AMENORRHEA

Edited by **Amar Chatterjee**

Amenorrhea
Edited by Amar Chatterjee

Published by InTech

Janeza Trdine 9, 51000 Rijeka, Croatia

Publishing Process Manager Iva Simcic

Technical Editor Teodora Smiljanic

Cover Designer InTech Design Team

Additional hard copies can be obtained from orders@intechopen.com

Amenorrhea, Edited by Amar Chatterjee
p. cm.
ISBN 978-953-307-988-2

For EU product safety concerns:
IN TECH d.o.o., Prolaz Marije Krucifikse Kozulić 3, 51000 Rijeka, Croatia,
info@intechopen.com or visit our website at intechopen.com.

Meet the editor

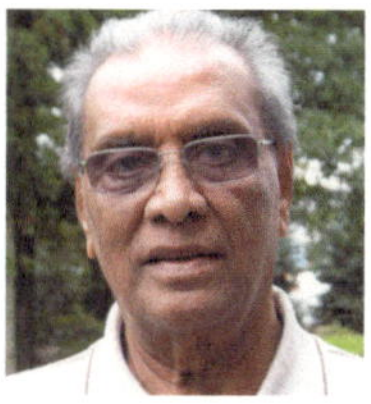

Professor Chatterjee obtained his Ph.D in 1966, Fellowship of Obstetrics & Gynaecology (FOG) in 1970 and was awarded the prestigious Doctor of Science (D.Sc) in 1976. He has been bestowed with numerous awards and honours that include Ford Foundation Fellowship, Fellow of the Zoological Society, Visiting Scientist (Ford Foundation), Fellow Malaysian Scientific Association, Honorary Postgraduate Lecturer (Calcutta University), Member of the International Editorial Board "Population Information", George Washington University Medical Centre (USA), Member of the Editorial Board of Biomedical Research and Research Career Development Award (FPF, India). Professor Chatterjee has published 127 original research articles in American, Canadian, European and other international journals. He has also presented several papers in national and international symposia. He is a member of the Society for the Study of Reproduction (USA), the Society for the Study of Fertlity (UK), the American Society of Andrology, the Physiological Society of India, the Zoological Society of India and the Malaysian Society of Pharmacology & Physiology.

Contents

Preface

This book is a wonderful collection of updated reviews by a group of experts dealing mostly with the aphysiological aspects of secondary amenorrhea.

The eight chapters of the book describe the hormonal evaluation of secondary amenorrhea, chemotherapy-related amenorrhea in breast cancer, a direct link between the nutritional status in anorectic women with amenorrhea and whether it is comparable with the thin postmenopausal women with risk of osteoporosis and fragility fracture. Other aspects include different lines of treatment of polycystic ovarian syndrome (PCOS)-related infertility and other problems. PCOS-associated insulin resistance, hyperinsulinemia with hyperandrogenism and their possible therapeutic interruption, the management of congenital adrenal hyperplasia-related insulin resistance and amenorrhea. It also covers clinical results of two new levenorgestrel-releasing intrauterine systems to reduce menstrual blood loss compared to surgical intervention. A review of literature and new insights on amenorrhea and endometrial ablation has also been described. The final chapter discusses the recent clinical application of campo (herbal) medicines for the treatment of amenorrhea.

Professor Dr Amar Chatterjee
Faculty of Medicine
Universiti Teknologi MARA
Shah Alam Campus, Selangor
Malaysia

1

Hormonal Diagnosis of Menstrual Irregularities or Secondary Amenorrhoea

Ursula Zollner
Department of Obstetrics and Gynecology
University of Würzburg
Germany

1. Introduction

In the daily clinical routine, clarification of menstrual irregularities is one of the major essentials for consultation in gynaecological practice. For an effective therapy, it is necessary to know the exact cause of the bleeding disorders. Menstrual irregularities can be the expression of a disturbed ovarian function or another disorder, usually uterine pathology. The type of menstrual irregularity is not necessarily indicative of the underlying disorder so that the examination of the levels of hormones is indispensable. Moreover, an organic cause of the bleeding disorder should be excluded. Whether the ovulatory cycle is associated with normal follicle maturation and corpus luteum function has to be clarified in the treatment of childlessness. The existence of anovulatory cycles or cycles with corpus luteum insufficiency can be normal in specific phases of life, e.g., puberty or peri-menopause. The issue of therapy should be addressed briefly. Firstly, the symptoms such as bleeding disorders and the disease patterns which are responsible for it should be highlighted. The clarification of menstrual irregularities is not only important in sterility therapy, they also influence the quality of life (1). Furthermore, hormonal disorders which are associated with chronic oestrogen or progesterone deficiency have an impact on the overall health (2). The following review represents the diagnostics of hormone-related menstrual irregularities in the fertile phase of life. The issue of bleeding disorders with the application of hormone preparations is not addressed.

2. Diagnostics of menstrual irregularities

Menstrual irregularities or bleeding disorders also include menstrual cycle-related symptoms such as dysmenorrhoea (1). During the classification of menstrual irregularities and/or bleeding disorders the only symptom which is assumed is bleeding, however, it does not contain any information about the cause of the deviation from regular menstrual cycles. A regular menstrual cycle with a 28-day bleeding interval in 85–90% of the cases is usually associated with normal ovarian function and corresponding ovulatory cycles (3). The normal bleeding duration is between 3–7 days and is associated with a blood loss of 30–40 ml (1). Deviations in the form of menstrual bleed which occur too infrequently or too frequently can be the expression of a pathological disorder. The causes can be uterine pathology, other illnesses or ovarian dysfunction. It can be assumed that 90% of all bleeding disorders are hormone-related or partly hormone-related (4). The menstrual irregularity can express itself through a change of the bleeding pattern (menstrual rhythm abnormalities), the intensity of bleeding, its duration (type of menstrual abnormalities) or in the form of additional bleedings. The bleeding disorders are to be interpreted with the age and/or the reproductive phase of the woman, respectively. An oligomenorrhoea in a 26-year-old obese patient is most likely to be due to a PCO syndrome. However, in a 46-year-old patient it probably indicates a perimenopausal condition. The physiological and/or the therapeutic menstrual irregularities must be disassociated from the pathological menstrual irregularities, e.g., the oligomenorrhoea in the perimenopause or the amenorrhoea under gestagen monotherapy.

3. Medical history

Whilst reviewing the medical history, all previous and current diseases (disorders of the liver or kidney function, autoimmune diseases) are inquired about. The current complaints, the medication (influence of prolactin production) and the questions concerning androgen-induced disorders are just as important questions as the questions concerning contraception, desire to have children or previous pregnancies. Lifestyle (sleep, physical activity) and eating habits must not be underestimated because endocrinological problems occur frequently in both overweight and underweight women as well as in the competitive athletes. Even extreme weight fluctuations can have an impact on the ovarian function. In this conjunction, the extremely important question concerns the coagulation dysfunctions because the execution of anticoagulation can influence the bleeding duration and intensity. Furthermore, questions should be asked about the presence of endocrinopathies such as diabetes mellitus (type I), Addison disease, Cushing disease, previous operation on the uterus and or the ovaries and/or operation or trauma of the pituitary area.

4. Menstruation history

During the medical history, attention should be paid to the exact increase in bleeding intervals. The patients often view their menstrual cycle is normal even if the intervals between them do not correspond to the standard of 24 to 34 days. However, a menstruation calendar can address the intervals, duration and the intensity of the bleeding. The estimation of the bleeding intensity is strongly influenced, therefore, number of sanitary towels and/or tampons per day is advised to be recorded. If lower abdominal pain is indicated then it is important to observe the temporal relation with the periods. A dysmenorrhoea can be a sentinel for an endometriosis. Premenstrual complaints such as headaches or mood swings can be the sign of premenstrual syndrome, an indication of corpus luteum insufficiency.

5. Clinical examinations

It is important to note that an acyclic vaginal bleeding does not always need to be an expression of a disturbed ovarian function. A large number of other factors, e.g., colpitis, ectopy, disturbed pregnancy or malignancies can become noticeable through a bleeding from the vagina and can often be diagnosed through the use of a speculum and/or a vaginal sonograpy. Physical and a gynaecological examination cannot be avoided during the diagnostic investigation of menstrual irregularities. The Body-Mass-Index, fat distribution pattern as well as androgen-induced disorders are very important, particularly in conjunction with the suspicion of PCO syndrome. During the gynaecological examination, infections, new formations or malformations of the internal genitals can be detected or excluded. Myomas, polyps or carcinomas should not be excluded as a cause for the bleeding. The vaginal sonography represents a substantial diagnosis test. By doing so, the condition and size of the uterus, endometrial thickness and the amount of layers as well as the form and the size of the ovaries can be assessed reliably. Follicular presence or absence is a good diagnostic criterion in assessing the egg cell reserve of the ovaries.

6. Hormonal diagnosis

Suspected diagnoses can usually be made through the type of the menstruation irregularity, symptoms and the results of the gynaecological examinations, which can then either be confirmed or excluded through a differentiated laboratory diagnosis. Therefore, an obese patient with secondary oligomenorrhoea and polycystic ovaries most likely suffers from PCO syndrome or a hyperandrogenemia. Conversely, a slim competitive athlete with a secondary amenorrhoea probably suffers from hypogonadotropic ovarian insufficiency. The menstrual phase must be taken into consideration when a blood sample is taken for investigation. It is proved to be useful to carry out the examination in the early follicle phase that is 3rd–5th days of menstruation. In secondary amenorrhoea, the question of selecting menstrual phase does not arise. The interpretation of hormones within the framework of the menstrual events implies the knowledge of the day of menstruation, the length of menstruation, the sequential secretion of the individual hormones during the course of a menstrual cycle and the relationship to one another (2, 8). The following hormones can be determined during the basic diagnostics (basic hormone analysis, [BHA], 3rd–5th days of the menstrual cycle). The following blood test should be done in a stress-free morning in early follicle phase:

- FSH (follicle-stimulating hormone)
- LH (luteinizing hormone)
- E_2 (estradiol)
- Progesterone
- Prolactin
- Testosterone
- Androstenedione
- DHEAS (dehydroepiandrosterone sulphate)
- 17-OH-Progesterone
- TSH (thyroid-stimulating hormone)

Depending on the assumed disease pattern, not all hormones need to be examined, rather it can be limited to the most relevant ones (see below). Table 1 shows the normal values of these hormones.

Hormone	Normal values
FSH	2 - 10 mIU/ml
LH	2 - 10 mIU/ml
Estradiol	25-200 pg/ml
Progesterone	< 1.0 ng/ml > 12 ng/ml in luteal hase
Prolactin	< 10 ng/ml
Testosterone	< 0.4 ng/ml
DHEAS	< 3.0 µg/ml
Androstendion	0.47–2.68 ng/ml
17-OH-Progesterone	0.2–1.0 ng/ml
TSH	0.2–3.5 µIU/ml

Table 1. Normal values of basic hormone analysis [BHA], 3rd–5th days of the menstrual cycle (3, 6)

7. Monitoring the menstrual cycle

If a largely inconspicuous menstrual rhythm is present, it is interesting in sterility diagnosis to see whether it really leads to ovulation or to a stable luteal phase. Follicle maturation disorder or corpus luteum insufficiency cannot be diagnosed through only one single blood test. Several examinations concerning the menstrual cycle are necessary. In this connection, the vaginal sonography can be implemented in addition to the laboratory diagnosis. One would expect the following values in such a diagnostic cycle:

- Day 3-5: BHA values are normal (see Table 1)
  Vaginal sonography: small endometrium , ovaries with a few
  small preantral follicles
- Day 12-14: LH normal or ↑, estradiol > 150 pg/ml
  Vaginal sonography: endometrium approx. 10 mm, mostly
  three-layered, dominant follicle approx. 16-20 mm
- Day 21: Progesterone > 10 ng/ml
  Vaginal sonography: endometrium approx. 10 mm, homogeneous,
  Corpus luteum with interior echoes

In the case of deviations, conclusion about the underlying disorder can be drawn. The carrying out of LH-urine tests for the determination of ovulation period which indicates the pre-ovulatory LH surge in the spontaneous menstrual cycle is in practice (5). Both the FSH levels and FSH/LH ratio (for values > 3.6 a reduced build up of follicles must be expected) as well as the AMH (Anti-Müller hormone) are used for evaluation of the ovarian reserve.

8. Practical approaches to the individual menstrual irregularity

In 1987, Hammerstein tried to classify the bleeding disorders according to their causes (9). This is how the functional (physiological) bleedings are differentiated from dysfunctional (hormonal cause) bleedings. Furthermore, iatrogenic (contraception, HRT) systemic

(systemic diseases such as coagulation disorders) bleedings are differed from organic (carcinoma, myoma, polyp) bleedings. Our suggestion is however, to classify the bleeding disorders according to the usual patterns and then to search for their causes (7). If a hormonal disorder is responsible instead of an organic disorder, the type of ovarian disorder can be defined more precisely, e.g., oligomenorrhoea in the case of PCO syndrome (WHO II) or secondary amenorrhoea in the case of hyperprolactinaemia (WHO VI). In the case of the following suggestions with regards to the practical approach, it is essential that an organic cause for the bleeding disorder (myoma, carcinoma, infection, coagulation disorder) has been excluded.

8.1 Primary amenorrhoea

The clarification of the primary amenorrhoea is not addressed here in greater detail. What is of greater importance than hormone diagnostics is the evaluation of secondary sexual characteristics. For example, if the breasts and pubic hair of a 17-year-old patient are normal it can be assumed that she has normal ovarian functions. In most cases a diagnosis (e.g., hymenal atresia or Mayer-Rokitansky-Küster syndrome) can be made through an exact evaluation of the internal sexual characteristics. If the secondary sexual characteristics are inadequately pronounced (infantile, virilised), a large number of diseases must be considered (delayed puberty, Turner syndrome, androgen receptor defects) whose clarification should at best be carried out in a special endocrinological consultation.

8.2 Secondary amenorrhoea

If the period fails to appear for more than three months although a spontaneous menstruation took place previously, then one speaks of a secondary amenorrhoea. It goes without saying that in this situation a pregnancy must be excluded. In order to prove at which level the disorder has occurred, the provision of the following hormone analysis should be adhered to:

- FSH, LH, estradiol, testosterone, androstendione, DHEAS, prolactin and TSH

At the same time, the sonographic image of the ovaries and the endometrium is relevant. The FSH, LH and estradiol values should be correlated with the sonographic image of the internal genitalia because the levels of the individual hormone are extremely variable on phases of the menstrual cycle and in the case of amenorrhoea one does not have a reference point for the last bleeding. In the case of increased FSH, LH and estradiol values for example, a highly established three-layered endometrium is present then one should rather think of a periovulatory than a perimenopausal situation. For the further diagnostic investigation, a menstrual cycle should be waited for or initiated (2).

8.3 Oligomenorrhoea

If possible, a basic diagnosis should be carried out on the 3rd–5th days of menstruation. The diagnostic investigation is not substantially different from the clarification in the case of the secondary amenorrhoea. Due to the clinically suspected PCO syndrome, the 17-OH-progesterone should also be codetermined. If it is increased, then a late-onset AGS (androgenital syndrome) can cause the symptoms. An ACTH test and a molecular-genetic clarification, if possible, would be necessary for further diagnostics.

- FSH, LH, estradiol, testosterone, androstendione, DHEAS, prolactin, 17-OH-progesterone and TSH
- If blood sampling is not possible in early follicle phase of the menstrual cycle, in addition, progesterone should be codetermined.

8.4 Polymenorrhoea

Most of the polymenorrhoeas are an expression of corpus luteum insufficiency, which in turn is due to a follicle maturation disorder. A normal luteal phase lasts for approx. 14 days, in case of duration of 10 days, an insufficient luteal phase can be assumed. Polymenorrhoeas however, can also occur in the case of a chronic anovulation as occurs in PCO syndrome. If a perimenopausal situation is present, one can limit it to the determination of FSH, LH and estradiol, otherwise a clarification as with oligomenorrhoea should take place.

- FSH, LH, estradiol, testosterone, androstendione, DHEAS, prolactin, 17-OH-progesterone and TSH
- Determination of progesterone in the mid-luteal phase for the demonstration of a corpus luteum insufficiency

8.5 Metrorrhagia and menorrhagia

In 30% of the cases, metrorrhagias have organic causes, 70% of the causes have to do with a dysfunctional bleeding which was triggered by persistent follicles or other hormonal disorders (1). Organic causes however include infections, myomas, carcinomas or coagulation disorders. Defining a bleeding disorder in a perimenopausal situation is difficult because it is often difficult to allocate it to one menstrual cycle (7). Metrorrhagias and menorrhagias often occur in the transitional phases such as puberty or perimenopause. If the progesterone challenge remains absent despite the high estradiol concentration as with the follicle persistence, the over-proliferated endometrium is rejected. A stepwise diagnostic investigation is recommended:

- FSH, LH, estradiol
- Determination of progesterone at mid-luteal phase for the demonstration of corpus luteum insufficiency
- Possible further search for the causes through a complete BHA

8.6 Supernumerary bleeding

All forms of the bleeding are referred to as 'supernumeray bleedings' which occur cyclically and in addition to the normal menstrual bleeding. A distinction is made between premenstrual, postmenstrual or ovulational bleeding depending on the time of its occurrence. These bleedings are also referred to as 'spitting', and its duration is less than three days. A premenstrual spotting is usually due to a relative progesterone deficiency, and a postmenstrual spotting can be indicative of a very low estradiol production. Both of these can be an expression of a follicle maturation disorder and/or the former can be due to corpus luteum insufficiency. An ovulational bleeding can be caused by a rapid post-ovulatory estradiol deficiency. Supernumerary bleedings can also be due to organic causes such as polyps, myomas, carcinomas, infections or coagulation disorders. If there is no desire to have children and if there is no strong indication of an endocrinopathy, a diagnostic investigation in the form of hormone analysis is not essential because a symptomatic therapy with a hormone preparation usually leads to the satisfaction of the patient.

8.7 Type of menstrual abnormalities

In the case of the differential diagnosis clarification of hypomenorrhoeas or hypermenorrhoea, it should be noted that heavier bleeding is often triggered by a uterus myomatosus or a long-term anticoagulation. If an organic and/or systemic cause is excluded, a symptomatic therapy is preferred. As a general rule, a hormone analysis is not necessary, except when there is the desire to have children.

9. Differentiation of ovarian dysfunctions

Menstrual irregularities (deviations from the regular four-week bleeding intervals) are usually accompanied by an ovulatory disorder so that one cannot consider the entities, menstrual irregularities and ovulational disorders separately. The bleeding disorder is the external sign that a possible disturbed ovarian function is present. The definition is purely descriptive (7). However, as has already been mentioned, other factors can be responsible for the deviation from normal menstrual cycle, e.g., infections or uterine causes. Uterine factors, such as myomas, are in turn favoured by hormonal imbalances so that here the transitions are fluent. If a disturbed ovarian function is present, an exact diagnosis could be made through laboratory determination of most of the important hormones. According to WHO, ovarian insufficiencies are classified in seven groups (7). To be specific, it relates to a classification of the amenorrhoeas. The individual endocrine disease pattern can also be reflected in menstrual rhythm abnormalities, such as oligomenorrhoeas or polymenorrhoeas. The exact knowledge of at what level the disorder is present is indispensible in order to be able to initiate an effective therapy.

10. Hypogonadotropic ovarian dysfunction

Hypogonadotropic amenorrhoea is usually functional (WHO Group I), with organic causes (Group VII) such as tumours or traumas are rare. A disturbed pulsatility of the GnRH secretion can lead to an insufficient FSH and LH production and consequently results in follicle maturation disorder. The causes for the functional disorder are extreme stress situations, such as anorexia nervosa, famines (war amenorrhoea) or intense physical exercise, such as competitive sports. An amenorrhoea is usually present but oligomenorrhoea is also possible.

10.1 Diagnostics

- Estimation of FSH, LH, estradiol, progesterone, prolactin, testosterone, androstendione, DHEAS and TSH:
  - Decreased gonadotropines, estradiol is also low.
  - A low level of progesterone points to a pre-ovulatory or ovarian dormancy.
  - To exclude hyperprolactinaemia and/or hyperandrogenaemia, determination of androgens and of prolactin should be considered.

  - TSH levels to exclude altered thyroid gland function.
- Due to suspected organic causes (additional symptoms such as headaches, impaired vision or dizziness and/or no functional cause for the hypogonadotropic situation) a MRT examination should be carried out.
- A GnRH test can be carried out in order to eliminate the possible hypothalamic or pituitary causes (3).

10.2 Therapy

In case of organic causes if necessary, an operation is indicated. In case of functional disorders, a causal treatment such as weight gain in the case of anorexia should be strived for if possible. In addition, in case of low estradiol levels, HRT should be indicated and if there is a desire to have children, hormonal stimulation should be indicated if necessary.

11. Hypergonadotropic ovarian dysfunction

WHO Group III represents the hypergonadotropic ovarian insufficiencies. If secondary oligomenorrhoea or amenorrhoea is present then (physiological) perimenopausal situation and/or premature failure of the ovarian function (age > 40) can be thought of (increased FSH and LH levels).

11.1 Diagnostics

- Determination of FSH, LH, estradiol, progesterone, prolactin, testosterone, androstendione, DHEAS and TSH:
  - FSH and/or LH are elevated, estradiol low
  - A low level of progesterone indicates a pre-ovulatory or ovarian dormancy
  - To exclude hyperprolactinaemia and/or hyperandrogenaemia as well as dysfunction of the thyroid gland, determination of androgens, prolactin and TSH is essential.
- Due to suspected POF, further diagnostic investigations (e.g., chromosome analysis to exclude Turner syndrome, search of autoimmune diseases or associated endocrinopathies) are essential.

11.2 Therapy

In case of young patients, there is an indication for hormone replacement therapy in order to avoid oestrogen-deficient situations. If there is a desire to have children, a hormonal stimulation with FSH can be tried depending on the starting situation, however, with little prospect for success.

12. Hyperprolactinaemia

Hyperprolactinaemic ovarian dysfunctions can be due to many causes. If the disorder is pronounced, an amenorrhoea can be present, in most cases however, there are menstrual irregularities such as oligomenorrhoeas or anovulatory eumenorrhoeas. If there is an ovarian insufficiency caused by prolactinoma it must be allocated to WHO Group V. The amenorrhoeas which are caused by drugs or other hyperprolatinaemic amenorrhoeas are allocated to WHO Group VI. Increased prolactin levels lead to an ovarian dysfunction through a disturbed GnRH pulsatility but also through an influence on the adrenal cortex in terms of inducing adrenocortical hyperandrogenaemia.

12.1 Diagnostics

- Determination of FSH, LH, estradiol, progesterone, prolactin, testosterone, androstendione, DHEAS and TSH:
  - Gonadotropins and estradiol are usually normal or decreased
  - Prolactin is increased, in case of values > 50 ng/ml an image diagnosis should be included.
  - An associated hyperandrogenaemia can occur
- Hypothyroidisms can lead to a hyperprolactinaemia through an increased release of TRH.
- To measure a latent hyperprolactinaemia (normal basic prolactin values) provocation tests such as metoclopramide test can be carried out.

12.2 Therapy

If possible, a causal therapy (changeover of medication) should be strived for, however, the treatment with dopamine agonists is indicated in most cases.

13. Hyperandogenaemic ovarian dysfunction

The most common form of hyperandrogenaemic ovarian dysfunction (WHO Group II) is represented by the PCO syndrome. Ovarian insufficiencies of WHO Group II include all disorders with normal FSH levels where the interplay of gonadotropins or other factors of the central ovarian regulation (with the exception of hyperprolactinaemia) is disturbed. One main part of this group creates the hyperandrogenaemic disorders (2). The PCO syndrome is not a disease per se, rather a complex comprised of several symptoms. According to the Rotterdam classification from 2003, two of the three criteria must be present so that the PCOS diagnosis can be made (10):

- Oligoovulation or anovulation
- Clinical and/or biochemical sign of hyperandrogenisation
- Polycystic ovaries and the exclusion of other causes (congenital adrenal hyperplasia, androgen producing tumours, Cushing disease).

In case of PCOS, different causes can lead to a similar disease pattern. The most common menstrual irregularity in case of PCO syndrome is represented by oligomenorrhoea. In case of insufficient follicle maturation, an amenorrhoea can also be present. Even polymenorrhoea is possible through follicular disorder without ovulation or with consecutive corpus luteum insufficiency.

13.1 Diagnostics

- Determination of FSH, LH, estradiol, progesterone, prolactin, testosterone, androstendione, DHEAS, 17-OH-progesterone and TSH:
  - LH/FSH > 1.5-2
  - Estradiol can be normal, decreased or even elevated
  - Hyperandrogenaemia, depending on the individual androgens, can be differentiated with the knowledge of their production areas (ovarian and adrenal hyperandrogenaemia).

- An ACTH test to exclude late onset AGS should take place if there is an increase of 17-OH-progesterone. A molecular genetic inspection can be carried out in the case of a striking ACTH test. The heterozygous form of 21 hydroxylase deficiency (most common cause for late-onset AGS) often remains latent during childhood. It manifests itself in women usually after puberty in the form of menstruation irregularities, androgenisation appearance or a PCO syndrome.

13.2 Therapy

Depending on the cause, living situation and symptoms, an antiandrogen ovulation inhibitor, ovarian stimulation with clomiphene, low dose FSH or corticosteroid treatment comes into question.

14. Corpus luteum insufficiency

Corpus luteum insufficiency relates to the normogonadotropic ovarian dysfunction. The cause for this is usually a follicle maturation disorder in the first half of the menstrual cycle which can lead to an insufficient formation of the corpus luteum. The luteal phase is shortened to less than 10 days so that it leads to a shortening of the cycle. Often premenstrual spotting is evident. The progesterone levels are too low. In the perimenopause phase, similar situation appears (physiological). However, the development of myomas or an endometriumperplasia, which in turn can aggravate the bleeding disorder, can be favoured through the relative progesterone deficiency. Corpus luteum insufficiency can be concomitant of other endocrine disorders. In case of a desire to have children, the cause should be carefully searched for.

14.1 Diagnostics

- Determination of progesterone in the mid-luteal phase (repeated > 10 ng/ml)
- For differential diagnosis BHA with FSH, LH, estradiol, prolactin, testosterone, androstendione, DHEAS and TSH are to be carried out:
  - FSH, LH and estradiol within the normal range
  - The determination of androgens, prolactin and TSH to be made to exclude hyperprolactinaemia and/or hyperandrogenaemia as well as dysfunction of the thyroid gland.
- If basal body temperature is managed (> 10 days of luteal phase).

14.2 Therapy

When planning to have children, an ovarian stimulation therapy can lead to an improved follicle maturation and more efficient formation of the corpus luteum.

15. Dysfunctions of the thyroid gland

Dysfunctions of the thyroid gland can lead to menstrual irregularities through the influence of the hypothalamic-pituitary system (WHO Group II). Hypothyroidism in particular is very important for gynaecological endocrinology. Clinical symptoms such as cold intolerance, reduced performance or dry, cold skin may confirm the diagnosis of hypothyroidism. Hyperthyroidism can become noticeable through heat intolerance, moist and warm skin or tachycardias. Menstrual irregularities can occur in both the circumstances.

15.1 Diagnostics

- Determination of FSH, LH, estradiol, progesterone, prolactin, testosterone, androstendione, DHEAS and TSH:
  - Hypothyroidism: TSH increased, hyperthyroidism: TSH decreased
  - Gonadotropins can be normal or depleted
  - Hyperprolactinaemia possible
  - Hyperandrogenaemia possible
- A TRH test should be carried out.

15.2 Therapy

If a dysfunction of the thyroid gland is diagnosed, dysfunction-related treatment should be installed and continued. In case of good thyroid function, repeated basal hormonal analysis is recommended.

16. Conclusion for the practice

Menstrual irregularities are usually contingent on ovarian dysfunction. The level of disorder can be identified after excluding organic causes through a basal hormonal analysis and thus an adequate therapy can be introduced. This chapter describes which hormones should be evaluated (11).

17. References

[1] Göretzlehner G., Göretzlehner U., Harlfinger W. Zur Nomenklatur der Zyklusstörungen. Frauenarzt 2005; 45: 34-37.

[2] Ludwig M. Systematische Differenzialdiagnostik der Amenorrhoe. Gynäkol Endokrinol 2006; 4: 39-51.

[3] Leidenberger F., Strowitzki T., Ortmann O. Klinische Endokrinologie für Frauenärzte. 3. Aufl., Springer Medizin Verlag Heidelberg 2005.

[4] Gaetje R., Kissler S., Scharl A. et al. Therapiemöglichkeiten der uterinen Blutungstörungen. Frauenarzt 2006; 47: 738-741.

[5] Steck T. Praxis der Fortpflanzungsmedizin. Schattauer-Verlag Stuttgart 2001.

[6] Schulte H.M., Ludwig M., Neumann G. Anabasis. 4. Aufl., Endokrinologikum Hamburg 2005.

[7] Feige A., Rempen A., Würfel W. et al. Frauenheilkunde. Urban und Schwarzenberg. Wien. Baltimore 1997.

[8] Silbernagl S, Despopoulos A. Taschenatlas der Physiologie. Thieme. Stuttgart. New York; 1988.

[9] Hammerstein J. Dysfunktionelle Blutungen - dyshormonale Blutungsstörungen. Arch Gynecol Obstet 1987; 242: 557-574.

[10] Feige A, Rempen A, Wurfel W, Caffier H, Jawny j. Frauenheilkunde. 1 Urban und 2 Schwarzenberg. Wien. Baltimore 1997. Strowitzki T. and von Wolff M. Polyzystisches Ovar-Syndrom - neue therapeutische Ansätze. Frauenarzt 2006; 47: 522-525.
[11] Zollner U, Dietl J. Hormondiagnostik von Zyklusstörungen - was ist sinnvoll? Gynäkologische Praxis 2010; 34: 267-282.

2

Chemotherapy-Related Amenorrhea in Breast Cancer: Review of the Main Published Studies, Biomarkers of Ovarian Function and Mechanisms Involved in Ovarian Toxicity

M. Berliere, F.P. Duhoux, Ch. Galant, F. Dalenc, J.F. Baurain, I. Leconte, L. Fellah, L. Dellvigne, P. Piette and J.P. Machiels
Catholic University of Louvain
Belgium

1. Introduction

Breast carcinoma is the most common cancer in women of reproductive age. In Europe and in the United States, approximately 30% of all breast cancers occur before menopause and 15% of women are diagnosed in the reproductive age (age of 45 or younger). Adjuvant chemotherapy prolongs disease-free survival (DFS) and overall survival (OS), especially in young women, but also induces long-term and severe side effects such as temporary or definitive ovarian function suppression which results in potential loss of fertility and premature exposure to the risks of menopause including cardiovascular diseases, osteoporosis, hot flashes and genitourinary dysfunctions Bines et al. (1996). The probability of menopause with chemotherapy depends on the type of regimen used and on the age of the patient. In the literature, the estimated risk of amenorrhea varies between 0% and 60% in women younger than 40 years and between 40% and 100% in women older than 40 years. Beyond age and the type of regimen used, important variations reflect different durations of follow-up and variable definitions of menopause and of chemotherapy-related amenorrhea Bines et al. (1996).

2. Defining menopause status

The average age of menopause in women of Caucasian/European origin is around 51 years Bines et al. (1996); Burger et al. (2007); Gracia et al. (2005); Welt et al. (2006). Pituitary gonadotrophins stimulate ovarian steroid hormone production (estrogens, progesterone and androgens). Estradiol [E2] Welt et al. (2006) and progesterone act via a negative feedback loop to inhibit pituitary gonadotrophin release. Hormone release occurs on a cyclical basis so that concentrations of follicle-stimulating hormone (FSH) peak in the mid-follicular phase and decrease during the luteal phase, rising again shortly before menstruation Randolph et al. (2006); Tanay & Fenton (2010). As E2 levels rise in the late follicular phase, concentrations of luteinizing hormone (LH) surge (via positive feedback) in mid-cycle and then fall again during the luteal phase (negative feedback) under the influence of progesterone and E2. Both

E2 and inhibin-B are under gonadotrophin influence. Both hormones are stimulated by FSH. This allows the preservation of E2 secretion in the late reproductive phase Randolph et al. (2006); Tanay & Fenton (2010); Welt et al. (2006). The decline in quality and quantity of ovarian follicles (ovarian aging process) Broekmans et al. (2009); Burger et al. (2008) triggers the hormonal and symptomatic changes of menopausal transition. This decline accelerates around age 35 when the number of oocytes drops to approximately 25,000 (having been approximately 300,000 at puberty). Anti-Müllerian hormone (AMH) Sowers et al. (2008); Yang et al. (2011) produced by small preantral follicles is one of the earliest markers of ovarian aging since it reflects the remaining pool of follicles. Compared with changes in FSH, LH, progesterone, AMH and inhibin-B secretions, the fall in E2 levels occurs relatively close to the menopause Welt et al. (2006). Before menopause, climacteric symptoms and bleeding irregularities can occur as a consequence of changes in E2 and progesterone secretion. Menopause is commonly defined as the last menstrual bleed or final menstrual period (commonly named FMP). This can only be recognized retrospectively after 12 consecutive months of amenorrhea. The FMP is typically preceded by a period of hormonal instability and irregularity in the menstrual cycle lasting up to several years. In the literature, there is no uniform definition of when this transitional period also called "perimenopause" begins.
However, different criteria (such as the first occurrence of more than 7 days difference in cycle length) have been proposed. Perimenopause extends until the 12 month-period of amenorrhea has elapsed. Prior to FMP, bleeding patterns are highly unpredictable, vasomotor symptoms are common but not present in all cases. There is no hormonal marker which infallibly signals permanent cessation of menstruation. In 2001, the stages of reproductive aging workshop proposed FSH Burger et al. (2007); Randolph et al. (2006) as the best marker available but did not establish levels that defined the menopause. FSH secretion itself is variable. Elevations may occur up to 10 years before the menopausal transition. Furthermore, there is a lack of agreement between assays, and body size and age have effects independent of menstrual status. Based on changes in menstrual cycles and levels of FSH, the first standardized classification of stages or reproductive aging workshop (STRAW) was proposed in 2001Soules et al. (2001). This classification includes 7 stages. These stages take into account not only the changes in bleeding patterns but also the changes in hormone levels. AMH could be of potential use in better defining the stages of menopausal transition. However, its widespread use has been precluded by cost and the lack of sensitivity and reproducibility of available assaysLedger (2010). According to the most recent National Comprehensive Cancer Network (NCCN) guidelines Guidelines (2010) on the management of breast cancer, a woman can reasonably be considered postmenopausal if any of the following conditions have been fulfilled :

- She has had prior bilateral oophorectomy.
- She is age 60 years or older.
- If less than 60, she has had amenorrhea of 1 year or longer in the absence of chemotherapy, tamoxifen, toremifene or ovarian suppression, and FSH and E2 levels are in the postmenopausal range.
- If she is taking tamoxifen or toremifene and is under 60 years of age, FSH and E2 levels are in the postmenopausal range.

The guidelines mention that it is not possible to determine menopausal status when a woman is taking a GnRH agonist or antagonist. If none of these conditions are fulfilled and yet the patient has infrequent or no menses, she should be considered pre- or perimenopausal.

3. Defining chemotherapy-related amenorrhea

In premenopausal patients, chemotherapy can induce temporary or permanent ovarian dysfunction Meirow (2000); Valagussa et al. (1993); Walshe et al. (2006).
The definition of CRA is not consistent across the literature and this helps explain the wide range in reported rates among chemotherapy trials Bines et al. (1996); Walshe et al. (2006). According to the American College of Obstetricans and Gynecologists, chemotherapy-related amenorrhea is defined as cessation of menses for 6 months. However other authors have defined CRA as the cessation of menses lasting 3 to 6 months or longer, or used the criterion of menstrual cessation lasting at least 12 months. Other difficulties are explained by the fact that inconsistencies exist in the way amenorrhea is reported. Some authors report the incidence of amenorrhea immediately upon completion of chemotherapy, while others select various time points after the start and end of chemotherapy Meirow (2000); Valagussa et al. (1993); Vegetti et al. (2000). The time point most commonly encountered in the literature is 12 months after the end of chemotherapy. Chemotherapy-related amenorrhea is generally linked to the patient's age as well as treatment protocol (types of chemotherapeutic agents used, doses and schedules) Bonadonna et al. (2005); Goldhirsch et al. (1990); Padmanabhan et al. (1986); Valagussa et al. (1993); Warne et al. (1973). Data on ovarian function are widely available for certain regimens, such as cyclophosphamide, methotrexate and 5-fluorouracil (CMF) polychemotherapy Bonadonna et al. (2005); Goldhirsch et al. (1990); Warne et al. (1973) and anthracycline-based treatments Hortobagyi et al. (1986); Levine et al. (1998); Pritchard et al. (2005); Roche et al. (2006), but fewer studies have been conducted on taxane-based regimens Abusief et al. (2006); Berlière et al. (2008); Clemons & Simmons (2007); Davis et al. (2005); Fornier et al. (2005); Martin et al. (2003; 2005); Tham et al. (2007), and they unfortunately show contradictory results. Other problems can be summarized by the lack of prospective studies and by the limited duration of follow-up.

4. Rates of chemotherapy-related amenorrhea with main cytotoxic agents

4.1 Cyclophosphamide-based regimens Bonadonna et al. (2005); Goldhirsch et al. (1990); Warne et al. (1973)

As previously mentioned, the incidence of ovarian dysfunction is related to patient age, the specific agents used and the total dose administered, especially the dose of alkyaling agents such as cyclophosphamide. Amenorrhea rates following combination chemotherapy consisting of CMF regimens range from 21% to 71% in women aged 40 years and younger, and from 40% to 100% in older ones Bonadonna et al. (2005); Goldhirsch et al. (1990); Padmanabhan et al. (1986); Warne et al. (1973). In the interpretation of the data with CMF regimens, many difficulties exist due to a lack of homogeneity of CMF regimens: variations in the doses and type of administration of cyclophosphamide (oral vs. intravenous) and variations in the total number of courses: 3 to 12 courses. In a manuscript dedicated to "30 years follow-up of randomized studies of adjuvant CMF in operable breast cancer", Bonadonna at al. Bonadonna et al. (2005) defined drug-induced amenorrhea as "the irreversible cessation of menstrual periods during chemotherapy treatment or in the first years of follow-up, in the absence of disease relapse". Amenorrhea rates were mentioned for 12 versus 6 cycles of CMF. CMF regimen consisted of cyclophosphamide (100 mg/m^2)/orally from day 1 to day 14, methotrexate (40 mg/m^2) intravenously on day 1 and 8, and 5-fluorouracil (600 mg/m^2) every 4 weeks. The incidence of iatrogenic amenorrhea was reported in the two regimens (6 cycles versus 12 cycles) by age group. Overall, drug-induced amenorrhea was reported more often in the longer regimen (75% versus 62%) than in the shorter one. In women younger than 45 years, the incidence of amenorrhea was 52.3% in the longer regimen vs. 31% in the shorter regimen. However, in women aged 45 or older, the incidence of amenorrhea was unrelated to the duration of treatment (97% vs. 96%). Unfortunately, only few investigators have considered the fact that chemotherapy may cause incomplete ovarian damage resulting in premature menopause months or years after completion of treatment.

4.2 Doxorubicin-based regimens Hortobagyi et al. (1986); Levine et al. (1998); Roche et al. (2006)

The association of doxorubicin with amenorrhea and infertility was initially debatableHortobagyi et al. (1986); Levine et al. (1998). Bines et al. Bines et al. (1996) reported an amenorrhea rate of 34% after therapy with adriamycin and cyclophosphamide (AC). However, these authors did not differentiate between younger and older women. A Canadian adjuvant trial (NCIC CTG MA5) Pritchard et al. (2005) that compared 6 courses of CMF (Standard Bonadonna regimen) (cyclophosphamide 100 mg/m^{2}orally days 1 through 15, methotrexate 40 mg/m^{2}Gracia et al. (2005) intraveinously days 1 and 8 and fluorouracil 60 mg/m^{2}Gracia et al. (2005) intraveinously days 1 and 8) with 6 courses of intensive CEF (cyclophosphamide 75 mg/m^{2}Gracia et al. (2005) orally days 1 through 14, epiadriamycin 60 mg/m^{2}Gracia et al. (2005) intraveinously days 1 and 8 and fluorouracil 500 mg/m^{2}intraveinously day 1 and 8) reported that the incidence of CRA was slightly higher in the CEF arm (51%) than in the CMF arm (42.6%). This difference was observed at 6 months but no difference was observed at 12 months. An interesting conclusion of this study is that late chemotherapy-induced amenorrhea (amenorrhea at 12 months) seems to be associated with improved outcome in premenopausal patients with receptor-positive breast cancer.

4.3 TaxanesAbusief et al. (2006); Berlière et al. (2008); Clemons & Simmons (2007); Davis et al. (2005); Fornier et al. (2005); Martin et al. (2003; 2005); Tham et al. (2007)

Taxanes, including paclitaxel and docetaxel, have recently been introduced in the adjuvant setting of breast carcinoma, based on Phase III data with adjuvant anthracycline and taxane combinations or sequences demonstrating significant benefits compared with non taxane-containing regimensClemons & Simmons (2007); Davis et al. (2005); Fornier et al. (2005); Martin et al. (2003); Roche et al. (2006); Tham et al. (2007). The rates of chemotherapy-induced amenorrhea associated with taxane-based regimens reported by different studies are discordant. Since taxanes are administered either sequentially or concurrently with anthracyclines and cyclophosphamide, it is difficult to evaluate the true impact of taxanes on the development of amenorrhea.

Breast Cancer International Research Group (BCIRG) Trial 001 Martin et al. (2003; 2005) reported an incidence of amenorrhea after adjuvant docetaxel 75 mg/m 2, doxorubicin 50 mg/m^{2}and cyclophosphamide 500 mg/m^2(TAC) 6 courses every 3 weeks or 5-fluorouracil 500 mg/m 2, doxorubicin 50 mg/m^{2}and cyclophosphamide 500 mg/m^2(FAC) of 51.4%

and 32.8%, respectively and the latest update of this trial presented at the San Antonio Breast Cancer Symposium in 2010 with a longer follow-up confirmed these results: 47% of amenorrhea in the TAC group versus 30% in the FAC group (median follow-up 10 years).
In the study by Fornier Fornier et al. (2005), 166 very young patients were reviewed. All patients were treated with AC (doxorubicin at a dose of 60 mg/m 2 + cyclophosphamide at a dose of 600 $mg/m^2$for 4 cycles followed by a taxane). The majority of patients were given AC followed by paclitaxel at a dose of 175 mg/m 2 for 4 cycles administered every 2 - 3 weeks. Only 7 patients received docetaxel (100 mg/m^2). In this cohort, long-term amenorrhea was defined as the absence of menstruations > 12 months after the completion of all chemotherapy. No hormone values were available and the conclusions of this study were that addition of a taxane did not appear to produce a higher rate of chemotherapy-related amenorrhea compared to historical controls.
In the study by Davis et al. Davis et al. (2005), 159 premenopausal patients were reviewed. As initial chemotherapy, 102 women received AC (doxorubicin - cyclophosphamide), 39 received CMF (cyclophosphamide – methotrexate-fluorouracil) and 18 received CAF (cyclophosphamide - doxorubicin - 5-fluorouracil). Following the initial regimen, 51 patients received additional adjuvant chemotherapy, generally with a taxane for 12 weeks (paclitaxel in 32 patients and docetaxel in 19 patients). The conclusions of this study were similar to those of Fornier et al. Fornier et al. (2005): sequential addition of taxanes did not appear to increase the risk of chemotherapy-induced amenorrhea, when added to a non-taxane regimen. Moreover, authors did not find any impact of the type of initial chemotherapy administered. Unfortunately, in this study, no hormone values were available.
More recently, Tham et al. Tham et al. (2007) published a study involving 191 patients (including 158 patients < 40 years of age at the start of chemotherapy). The patients received 4 cycles of AC alone or followed by a taxane. There was no stratification between paclitaxel and docetaxel. The definition of CRA was a little different in this study. Indeed, it was defined as cessation of menses within 1 year of starting chemotherapy and lasting > 6 months.
In a subgroup of young patients (< 40 years), addition of a taxane resulted in a higher incidence of CRA (61% versus 44%). In women over 40 years of age, amenorrhea rates were high in both the group of AC alone and the group of AC followed by a taxane (81% versus 85%). No statistically significant difference was observed between the two groups.
Our team and the team of Toulouse Berlière et al. (2008); Roche et al. (2006) conducted a substudy with patients included in the PACS 01 study. The main objective of our retrospective study was to evaluate the incidence of reversible chemotherapy-related amenorrhea in patients treated with 6FEC (5-fluorouracil 500 mg/m^2, epirubicin 100 $mg/m^2$and cyclophosphamide 500 mg/m^2) and 3FEC/3D (3 FEC followed by 3 docetaxel 100 mg/m 2), and the impact of sequential docetaxel on the rate of CRA. The incidence of CRA at the end of chemotherapy was similar in the 2 groups: 93% in the 6FEC arm and 92.8% in the 3FEC/3D arm. However, in the year following the end of chemotherapy, more patients recovered menses in the 3FEC/3D arm than in the 6FEC arm: 35% versus 23.7% (p=0.019). Among the patients for whom hormone values were available, 43% in the 3FEC/3D arm and 29% in the 6FEC arm showed premenopausal levels one year after the end of chemotherapy (p<0.01).

5. Prognostic impact of chemotherapy-related amenorrhea

Whether or not induction of amenorrhea by cytotoxic chemotherapy (34-44) is a prognostic factor in the treatment of premenopausal women is still controversial. A positive impact on DFS was found by some Aebi et al. (2000); Borde et al. (2003); Brincker et al. (1987); Del Mastro et al. (1997); Parulekar et al. (2005); Poikonen et al. (2000); Powles (1998); Swain et al. (2010) but not confirmed by others Ferretti et al. (2006); Vanhuyse et al. (2005). Del Mastro et al Del Mastro et al. (1997) conducted a review of 13 studies involving 3929 patients undergoing CMF-based regimens, with follow- up ranging from 3 to 20 years. A statistically significant association was found between the development of chemotherapy-related amenorrhea and DFS. In the majority of cases, OS was found to be associated with amenorrhea (in 3 out of 5 studies reviewed). In a study recently published by Parulekar et al. Parulekar et al. (2005), similar results were observed with intensive CEF (cyclophosphamide, epirubicin, 5-fluorouracil therapy), which induced a higher rate of amenorrhea than the classic CMF protocol, but OS was also better in the CEF arm than in the CMF arm.
In the Trial VI study by the International Breast Cancer Study Group (IBCSG)Goldhirsch et al. (1990) cessation of menses, even for a limited time period, appeared to be beneficial, especially in patients with ER-positive breast tumors. In this study, however, the greatest effect was observed in patients receiving suboptimal treatment with only 3 initial CMF courses. Bonadonna et al.Pagani et al. (1998) exhibits a different point of view. Their analysis of the influence of drug-induced amenorrhea on the therapeutic outcome after CMF treatment refutes the hypothesis that adjuvant chemotherapy acts merely as chemical castration. As reported in many individual trials and the worldwide overview, adjuvant chemotherapy benefits hormone-responsive and hormone-unresponsive tumors, whereas endocrine therapy has no worthwhile benefit in E2 receptor-negative subpopulations. Bonadonna et al. Bonadonna et al. (2005) estimates that adjuvant chemotherapy has cytotoxic effects regardless of the putative hormone dependency of the tumor cells.
In the PACS 01 trial Roche et al. (2006), a survival advantage in favor of the 3FEC/3D arm was observed only for women aged over 50 years, but not for the younger population. The reason for this is unclear but the impact of reversible amenorrhea needs to be investigated further, since our small retrospective analysis suggests that amenorrhea Berlière et al. (2008) was correlated with DFS in the 3FEC/3D group. In the NSABP B30 trialGanz et al. (2011), 5531 breast cancer patients were randomly assigned to sequential doxorubicin (A) 20 mg/m 2 + cyclophosphamide (C) 600 mg/m 2 4 courses every 3 weeks followed by docetaxel (T) 100 mg/m^{2}4 courses every 3 weeks, or concurrent TAC (docetaxel 75 mg/m^2, doxorubicin 50 mg/m^{2}and cyclophosphamide 500 mg/m^{2}4 courses every 3 weeks) or 4 cycles of AT (doxocuribin 50 mg/m 2 + docetaxel 75 mg/m 2 every 3 weeks). Tamoxifen was administered in all patients with E2 hormone receptor positive tumors. The results indicated that patients with more than 6 months amenorrhea had a better prognosis than patients with a shorter period of amenorrhea.

6. Assessing post-chemotherapy ovarian function

Assessing post-chemotherapy ovarian function in breast cancer survivors of late reproductive age is important to clinical decision making on a range of issues such as choice of endocrine therapy Berlière et al. (2010); Ganz et al. (2011); Su (2010). It is therefore important to analyze the different available tools.

Currently, the primary tool for assessing post-chemotherapy ovarian function is menstrual pattern. However, in patients who received chemotherapy and endocrine therapy, lack of menses does not always represent ovarian failure.
In an abstract presented in poster form at the San Antonio Breast Cancer Symposium in 2010 Berlière et al. (2010), we reported the results of a prospective study conducted in our Breast Clinic between 1999 and 2003, comparing ovarian function between premenopausal breast cancer patients receiving tamoxifen alone (group I) and those receiving tamoxifen following chemotherapy (group II). 138 premenopausal patients, treated for early breast cancer were included: 68 patients in the group of tamoxifen alone and 70 patients in the group of tamoxifen administered after chemotherapy (6 cycles of FEC 100 on day 1 every 3 weeks – 5- fluorouracil 500 mg/m^2, epirubicin 100 mg/m^{2}and cyclophosphamide 500 mg/m 2 – or 4 cycles of EC on day 1 every 3 weeks – epiadriamycin 75 mg/m 2 and cyclophosphamide 500 mg/m^2). All patients had a confirmed premenopausal status (biological data) at the entry of the study or 3 months later. Three patients were out of study in groups I and 2 were out of study in group II. The results of this prospective study were analyzed at the end of 2009. We identified 4 different ovarian patterns of response to tamoxifen in the 2 groups:

1. regular menses (> 10 cycles/year)
2. oligomenorrhea (5 to 9 cycles/year)
3. severe oligomenorrhea(1 to 4 cycles/year)
4. complete amenorrhea.

The number of patients in each subgroup was respectively

- for group I (65 patients): 3 (4%), 19 (29%), 38 (58%) and 5 (8%)
- for group II (68 patients): 2 (3%), 21 (30%), 38 (55%) and 7 (10%).

We confirmed that amenorrhea is an insufficient parameter to define menopausal status in patients receiving tamoxifen. The most common biomarkers used are FSH and E2. Low E2 levels are also insufficient to define menopause because while on tamoxifen therapy patients can exhibit low E2 levels, low FSH levels and oligomenorrhea. These data are very important in the choice of endocrine therapy.
Measurement of ovarian reserve in breast cancer survivors may increase understanding of a woman's reproductive potential after cancer chemotherapy Partridge et al. (2008; 2010); Su (2010). Reproductive potential is generally related both to the quantity and quality of ovarian primordial follicles. Several other markers of ovarian reserve have been evaluated including early follicular phase serum E2, FSH, AMH and inhibin-B as well as measurements of antral follicle count (AFC) and ovarian volume. The interesting study of Partridge et al. Partridge et al. (2010) confirms that young breast cancer survivors who have undergone cytotoxic chemotherapy and remain premenopausal have diminished AFC levels when compared with healthy controls. This study also reveals that a lower level of AMH appears to be the best serum predictor of diminished AFC Partridge et al. (2008; 2010), which is thought to reflect reduced likelihood of future pregnancy. AMH, the anti-Müllerian hormone, is a member of the transforming growth factor β (TGFβ) family and is produced by FSH-sensitive early antral follicles. In this way, it may be a more sensitive predictor of ovarian reserve than other markers, such as AFC and inhibin-B, which detect more mature primordial follicles. Some studies exhibit interesting results Anderson & Cameron (2011); Domingues et al. (2010); Knauff et al. (2009); Rosendahl et al. (2010); Yu et al. (2010). In the study of

Partridge Domingues et al. (2010); Partridge et al. (2010), AFC and AMH seem to be the best markers of ovarian reserve. These two markers are highly correlated and for breast cancer patients receiving tamoxifen, lower AFC, AMH and inhibin-B were observed than for non-tamoxifen-treated survivors.
However, it is important to insist on the fact that breast cancer survivors can become pregnant with undetectable levels of AMH Anderson & Cameron (2011). In our institution, this year and the year before, 4 patients (30, 39, 36 and 30 years respectively) became pregnant with undetectable levels of AMH, but we have no values before the start of chemotherapy. Some variations of AMH while on metformin, tamoxifen and aromatase inhibitors have been described Cordes et al. (2010); Dieudonné et al. (2011); Panidis et al. (2010).
In conclusion, AMH seems to be the most interesting biological marker but further prospective studies are needed to evaluate the exact value of the different markers (AFC, AMH and inhibin-B). In the future, women interested in post-treatment fertility may be able to undergo ovarian reserve testing before and upon completion of systemic therapy. Prospective studies are needed to determine the predictive values of these tests for pregnancy after chemotherapy as well as the potential value in predicting premature menopause in young cancer survivors. Quality of life outcomes also need to be investigated prospectively Knobfm (2006).

7. Mechanisms of ovarian injury

The follicular reserve within the ovaries consists mainly of quiescent primordial follicles developed during fetal life. A tremendous number of primordial follicles will be annihilated before or shortly after birth and throughout postnatal life by a physiological programmed cell death process named apoptosis Faddy & Gosden (1995). This physiological cellular machinery may predispose the follicles to apoptosis induced by exogenous signals, such as chemotherapeutic agents. The first histological study performed on human ovaries after chemotherapy Browne et al. (2011); Meirow et al. (2007; 1999) demonstrated that the end result of chemotherapy was ovarian atrophy and global loss of primordial follicles. But the effect of chemotherapy on the ovary is not an "all or nothing phenomenon". The mechanisms involved in the loss of primordial follicles in response to anticancer therapy are not well understood. A few human and animal studies Faddy & Gosden (1995); Meirow et al. (1999) demonstrated that chemotherapy-induced damage to ovarian pregranulosa cells and that apoptosis occurred during oocyte and follicle loss.
The results of a study conducted by Meirow et al. Meirow et al. (2007) indicate that injury to blood vessels and focal fibrosis of the ovarian cortex are present in ovaries of patients previously exposed to chemotherapy. These modes of injury were present in non-atrophic ovaries of patients that were not sterilized by chemotherapy.
Ben Aharon and his coworkers Ben-Aharon et al. (2010) evaluated the effects of doxocuribin (injected intraperitoneally) on mice ovaries. A single injection of doxorubicin resulted in a major reduction in both ovarian size and weight that lasted even one month post-treatment. A dramatic reduction in ovulation rate was also observed one week after treatment, followed by a partial recovery at one month. In an attempt to characterize the apoptotic effect of doxorubicin on the ovary, the authors were able to detect apoptosis in histological sections of mice ovaries by depicting caspase-3 activity and TUNEL staining. The authors observed in the doxorubicin-treated mice a loss of premature follicles as well as perivascular changes already

described in human ovaries following administration of other chemotherapeutic agents such a cyclophosphamide and cisplatin Browne et al. (2011); Meirow et al. (1999).
In a study conducted in our laboratory, mice were injected intraperitoneally with a single dose of cyclophosphamide (200 mg/kg). These experiments did not allow us to identify an increase of apoptosis in mice ovaries treated with cyclophosphamide.
Other previous studies also showed that a single dose of cyclophosphamide was not associated with an increased rate of apoptosis. This is why in our laboratory, we will repeat the injections of cyclophosphamide in new experiments to try to observe apoptosis in mice ovaries.
The studies of Meirow et al. Meirow et al. (2007) and Aharon Ben-Aharon et al. (2010) hypothesized a combined mechanism of neovascularization and ovarian tissue scarring with a direct toxic effect on the primordial follicles.
Personally, we think that additional processes that lead to ovarian damage and follicles loss after chemotherapy may be involved such as vascular complications and ischemic mechanisms. We have also planned to investigate these mechanisms on mice ovaries. Other drugs such as taxanes need also to be studied to elucidate ovarian toxicity of modern drugs and to give accurate information to young breast cancer patients.

8. Conclusion

This chapter was written after review of the literature (Pubmed research) and after analysis of personal data (PACS 01 substudy, evaluation of ovarian function while on tamoxifen, personal laboratory experiments). Our review highlights important difficulties:

- The definition of chemotherapy-related amenorrhea suffers from a lack of uniformity in the literature.
- Many studies are retrospective and evaluate old chemotherapy regimens. In the prospective studies, the duration of follow-up is too short and very often limited to anamnestic data.
- We thus recommend a prospective evaluation of endocrine function before chemotherapy and after treatment completion, and in this context we have initiated a multicentric prospective study. Follow-up has to last for a very long time (10 years minimum).
- The impact of taxanes on ovarian function requires further studies and laboratory studies.

Correct estimation of the risk of menopause and possibilities for preserving fertility according to age and treatment will facilitate the decision-making process regarding adjuvant therapy in breast cancer. This process requires precise information and will enable each patient to balance the potential benefits of treatment against the potential adverse effects and future risk.

9. References

Abusief, M., Missmer, S., Ginsburg, Weeks, J., Wiener, E. & Partridge, A. (2006). The effect of paclitaxel, dose density and trastuzumab in chemotherapy-related amenorrhea (cra) in premenopausal women with breast cancer, *San Antonio* p. Abstract 2079.

Aebi, S., Gelbert, S., Castiglione-Guertsh, M., Gelbert, R., Collins, J., Thürlimann, B., Rudenstam, C., Lindtner, J., Crivellari, D., Cortes-Funes, H., Simoncini, E., Werner, I., Coates, A. & Goldhirsch, A. (2000). Is chemotherapy alone adequate for young women with estrogen receptor-positive breast cancer?, *Lancet* 355: 1869–1874.

Anderson, R. & Cameron, D. (2011). Pretreatment serum Anti-müllerian hormone predicts long- term ovarian function and bone mass after chemotherapy for early breast cancer, *J Clin Endocrinol Metab* 96(5): 1333–43.

Ben-Aharon, I., Bar-Joseph, H., Tzarfaty, G., Kuchinsky, L., Eizel, S., Stemmer, S. & Shalbi, R. (2010). Doxorubicin-induced ovarian toxicity, *Reprod Biol Endocrinol* 8: 20.

Berlière, M., Dalenc, F., Malingret, N., Vindevogel, A., Pierre, P., Roche, H., Donnez, J., Symann, M., Kerger, J. & Machiels, J. (2008). Incidence of reversible amenorrhea in women with breast cancer undergoing adjuvant anthracyclin-based chemotherapy with or without docetaxel, *BMC Cancer* 8: 56.

Berlière, M., Dalenc, F., Piquard, N., Leconte, I., Fellah, L., Baurain, J., Galant, C., Duhoux, F. & Machiels, J. (2010). Tamoxifen and ovarian function, *San Antonio,* Abstract n°9544-13.

Bines, J., Oleske, D. & Cobleigh, M. (1996). Ovarian function in premenopausal women treated with adjuvant chemotherapy for breast cancer., *J Clin Oncol* 14: 1718–1729.

Bonadonna, G., Moliterni, A., Zambetti, M., Daidone, M., Pilotti, S., Gianni, L. & Valagussa, P. (2005). 30 years' follow-up of randomised studies of adjuvant CMF in operable breast cancer, *BMJ* p. BMJ 10.1136/BMJ 38314. 6220958F.

Borde, F., Chapelle-Marcilac, I., Fumoleau, P., Hery, M. & Roché, H. (2003). Role of chemotherapy- induced amenorrhea in premenopausal node-positive operable breast cancer patients: 9-year follow-up results of french adjuvant study group, *FASG data base. Breast Cancer Res Treat* 1982, S30.

Brincker, H., Rose, C., Rank, F., Mouridsen, H., Jacobsen, A., Dombernowsky, P., Panduro, J. & Andersen, K. (1987). Evidence of a castration-mediated effect of adjuvant cytotoxic chemotherapy in premenopausal breast cancer, *J Clin Oncol* 5: 1771–1778.

Broekmans, L., Soules, M. & Fauser, B. (2009). Ovarian aging: mechanisms and clinical consequences, *Endoc Rev* 30(5): 463–93.

Browne, H., Moon, K., Mumford, S., Schisterman, E., Decherney, A., Segars, G. & Armstrong, A. (2011). Anti-müllerian marker of acute cyclophosphamide-induced ovarian follicular destruction in mice pretreated with cetrorelix, *Fertil Steril* .

Burger, H., Hale, G., Dennerstein, L. & Robertson, D. (2008). Cycle and hormone changes during perimenopause: the key role of ovarian function, *Menopause* 15(4): 603–12.

Burger, H., Hale, G., Robertson, D. & Dennerstein, L. (2007). A review of hormonal changes during the menopausal transition: focus on findings from the melbourne women's midlife health project., *Hum Reprod Update* 13: 559–65.

Clemons, M. & Simmons, C. (2007). Identifying menopause in breast cancer patients: considerations and implications, *Breast Cancer Res. Treat.* 104: 115–120.

Cordes, T., Schultz-Mosgau, A., Diedrich, K. & Griesinger, G. (2010). Ongoing pregnancy after human menopausal gonadotrophin stimulation and timed intercourse in 40 years old women with undetectable Anti-müllerian hormone levels, *Fertil Steril* 94(4): e71–2.

Davis, L., Klitus, M. & Mintzer, D. (2005). Chemotherapy-induced amenorrhea from adjuvant breast cancer treatment: the effect of the addition of taxanes, *Clin. Breast Cancer* 6(5): 421–424.

Del Mastro, L., Venturini, M., Sertoli, M. & Rosso, R. (1997). Amenorrhea induced by adjuvant chemotherapy in early breast cancer patients: prognostic role and clinical implications, *Breast Cancer Res Treat* 43: 189–190.

Dieudonné, A., Vandenberghe, J., Geerts, I., Billen, J., Paridaens, R., Wildiers, H. & Neven, P. (2011). Undectable Anti-müllerian hormone levels and recovery of chemotherapy-induced ovarian failure in women with breast cancer on an oral aromatase inhibitor, *Menopause* p. 12.

Domingues, T., Rocha, A. & Serafini, P. (2010). Test for ovarian reserve: reliability and utility, *Curr Opin Obstet Gynecol* 22(4): 271–6 (review).

Faddy, M. & Gosden, R. (1995). A mathematical model of follicle dynamics in the human ovary, *Hum Reprod* 10: 770–5.

Ferretti, G., Carlini, P., Bria, E., Felici, A., Giannarelli, D., Ciccarese, M., Papaldo, P., Fabi, A. & Cognetti, F. (2006). Chemotherapy-induced amenorrhea in early breast cancer, *Ann Oncol* 17(2): 352.

Fornier, M., Modi, S., Panageas, K., Norton, L. & Hudis, C. (2005). Incidence of chemotherapy-induced, long-term amenorrhea in patients with breast carcinoma aged 40 years and younger after adjuvant anthracycline and taxane, *Cancer* 104(8): 1575–1579.

Ganz, P., Land, S., Geyer, C. J., Scecchini, R., Costantino, J., Pajon, E., Fehrenbacher, L., Atkins, J., Polikoff, J., Vogel, V., Erban, J., Livingston, R., Perez, E., Mamounas, E., Wolmark, N. & Swain, M. (2011). Menstrual history and quality of life outcomes in women with node positive breast cancer treated with adjuvant therapy in the NSABP B30 trial, *J Clin Oncol* 29(9): 1110–16.

Goldhirsch, A., Gelber, R. & Castiglione, M. (1990). The magnitude of endocrine effects of adjuvant chemotherapy for premenopausal breast cancer patients: the international breast cancer study group, *Ann Onco* 1: 183–188.

Gracia, C., Sammel, M., Freeman, E., Lin, H., Langan, E., Kapoor, S. & al (2005). Defining menopause status: creation of a new definition to identify the early changes of the menopausal transition., *Menopause* 12: 128–35.

Guidelines (2010). Breast cancer NCC and practice guidelines in oncology.

Hortobagyi, G., Buzdar, A., Marcus, C. & Smith, T. (1986). Immediate and long-term toxicity of adjuvant chemotherapy regimens containing doxorubicin in trials at M.D Anderson hospital and tumor institute, *J Natl Cancer Inst Monogr* 1: 105–109.

Knauff, E., Eijkemans, N., Lambalk, C., ten Kate-Booij, N., Hoek, A., Beerendonk, C. & Fauser, B. e. a. (2009). Anti-müllerian hormone, inhibin-b and antral follicles count in young women with ovarian failure, *Dutch Premature Ovarian Failure Consortium. J Clin Endocrinol Metab* 94(3): 786–92.

Knobfm, T. (2006). The influence of endocrine effects of adjuvant therapy on quality of life outcomes in younger breast cancer survivors, *The Oncologist* 11: 96–110.

Ledger, W. (2010). Clinical utility of measurement of Anti-müllerian hormone in reproductive endocrinology, *J Clin Endocrinol Metab* 95(12): 5144–54.

Levine, M., Brawell, V., Pritchard, K., Norris, B., Shepherd, L., Abu-Zahra, H., Findlay, B., Warr, D., Bowman, D., Myles, J., Arnold, A., Vandenberg, T., Mackenzie, R., Robert, J., Ottaway, J., Burnell, M., Williams, C. & Tu, D. (1998). Randomized trial of intensive cyclophosphamide, epirubicin and fluorouracil chemotherapy compared with cyclophosphamide, methotrexate and fluorouracil in premenopausal women with node- positive breast cancer, *National Cancer Institute of Canada. Clinical Trial School. J Clin Oncol* 16: 2651–2658.

Martin, M., Pienkowski, T., Mackey, J., Pawlicki, M., Guastalla, J., Weaver, C., Tomiak, E., Al-Tweigeri, T., Chap, L., Juhos, E., Guevin, R., Owell, A., Fornander, T., Hainsworth, J., Coleman, R., Vinholes, J., Modiano, M., Pinter, T., Tang, S., Colwell, B., Prady, C., Provencher, L., Walde, D., Rodriguez-Lescure, A., Hugh, J., Loret, C., Rupin, M., Blitz,

S., Jacobs, P., Murawsky, M., Riva, A. & Vogel, C. (2003). TAC improves disease-free survival and overall survival over FAC in node-positive early breast cancer patients, BCIRG 001, *SABCS* .

Martin, M., Pienkowski, T., Mackey, J., Pawlicki, M., Guastalla, J., Weaver, C., Tomiak, E., Al-Tweigeri, T., Chap, L., Juhos, E., Guevin, R., Owell, A., Fornander, T., Hainsworth, J., Coleman, R., Vinholes, J., Modiano, M., Pinter, T., Tang, S., Colwell, B., Prady, C., Provencher, L., Walde, D., Rodriguez-Lescure, A., Hugh, J., Loret, C., Rupin, M., Blitz, S., Jacobs, P., Murawsky, M., Riva, A. & Vogel, C. (2005). Adjuvant docetaxel for node-positive breast cancer, *N Engl J Med* 352(22): 2302–12.

Meirow, D. (2000). Reproduction post-chemotherapy in young cancer patients, *Mol Cel Endocrinol* 169: 123–131.

Meirow, D., Kaufman, B., Shrim, A., Rabinovici, J., Schiff, L., Raanani, H., Lebron, J. & Fridman, E. (2007). Cortical fibrosis and blood-vessels damage in human ovaries exposed to chemotherapy: potential mechanisms of ovarian injury, *Hum Reprod* 22: 1626–33.

Meirow, D., Lewis, H., Nugent, D. & Epstein, M. (1999). Subclinical depletion of primordial follicular reserve in mice treated with cyclophosphamide: clinical importance and proposed accurate investigative tool, *Hum Reprod* 14: 1903–07.

Padmanabhan, N., Howell, A. & Rubens, R. (1986). Mechanism of action of adjuvant chemotherapy in early breast cancer, *Lancet* 2: 411–414.

Pagani, O., O'Neill, A., Castiglione, M., Gelber, R., Goldhirsch, A., Rudenstam, C., Lindtner, J., Collins, J., Crivellari, D., Coates, A., Cavalli, F., Thürlimann, B., Simoncini, E., Fey, M., Price, K. & Senn, H. (1998). Prognostic impact of amenorrhea after adjuvant chemotherapy in premenopausal breast cancer patients with axillary node involvement: results of the international breast cancer study group (IBCSG) trial VI, *Eur J Cancer* 34(5): 632–640.

Panidis, D., Geopoulos, N., Piouka, A., Katsikis, I., Saltamavros, A., Devalas, G. & Diamanti-Kandarakis, E. (2010). The impact of oral contraceptives and metformine on Anti-müllerian hormone serum levels in women with polycystic ovari syndrome and biochemical hyperandrogenemia, *Gynecol Endocrinol* p. 14.

Partridge, A., Gelber, S., Peppercorn, J., Ginsburg, E., Sampson, E., Rosenberg, Przypyszny, M. & Winger, E. (2008). Fertility and menopausal outcomes in young breast cancer survivors, *Clin Breast Cancer* 8: 65–9.

Partridge, A., Ruddy, K., Gelber, S., Schapira, L., Abusief, M., Meyer, M. & Ginsburg, E. (2010). Ovarian reserve in women who remain premenopausal after chemotherapy for early stage breast cancer, *Fertil Steril* 94(2): 638–44.

Parulekar, W., Day, A., Ottaway, J., Shepherd, L., Trudeaun, M., Bramwell, V., Levine, M. & Pritchard, K. (2005). Incidence and prognostic impact of amenorrhea during adjuvant therapy in high-risk premenopausal breast cancer: analysis of a national cancer institute of canada clinical trials group study / NCIC CTG MA.5, *J Clin Oncol* 23: 6002–6008.

Poikonen, P., Saarto, T., Elomaa, I., Joensuu, H. & Blomqvist, C. (2000). Prognostic effect of amenorrhea and elevated serum gonadotrophin levels induced by adjuvant chemotherapy in premenopausal node-positive breast cancer patients, *Eur J Cancer* 36: 43–48.

Powles, T. (1998). Prognostic impact of amenorrhea after adjuvant chemotherapy, *Eur J Cancer* 34: 603–605.

Pritchard, K., Levine, M., Bramwell, V., Shepherd, L., Tu, D. & Paul, N. (2005). A randomised trial comparing CEF to CMF in premenopausal women with node positive breast cancer. update of NCIC CGT MA5 (national cancer institute of canada clinical trials group trial MA5), *J. Clin. Oncol* 23(22): 5166–70.

Randolph, J., Crawford, S., Dennerstein, L., Cain, K., Harlow, S., Little, R., Mithcell, E., B, N., Taffe, J. & Yosef, M. (2006). The value of follicle-stimulating hormone concentration and clinical findings as markers of the late menopausal transition., *J Clin Endocrin Metab* 91: 3034–40.

Roche, H., Fumoleau, P., Spielmann, M., Canon, J., Delozier, T., Serin, D., Symann, M., Kerbrat, P., Soulié, P., Eichler, F., Viens, P., Monnier, A., Vindevoghel, A., Campone, M., Goudier, M., Bonneterre, J., Ferrero, J., Martin, A., Geneve, J. & Asselain, B. (2006). Sequential adjuvant epirubicin-based and docetaxel chemotherapy for node-positive breast cancer patients: the FNLCC PACS 01 trial, *J Clin Oncol* 24: 5664–5671.

Rosendahl, M., Andersen, C., La Cour Freiesleben, N., Juul, A., Loss, K. & Andersen, A. (2010). Dynamics and mechanisms of chemotherapy-induced ovarian follicular depletion in women of fertile age, *Fertil Steril* 94(1): 156–66.

Soules, M., Sherman, S., Parrott, E., Rebar, R., Santoro, N., Utian, W. & Woods, N. (2001). Stages of reproductive aging workshop (STRAW), *J Women's Health Gend Based Med* 10: 843–8.

Sowers, M., Eyvazzadeh, A., Mc Connell, D., Yosef, M., Jannausch, M., Zhang, D., Harlow, S. & Randolph, J. (2008). Anti-müllerian hormone and inhibin-b in the definition of ovarian aging and the menopause transition, *J Clin Endocrinol Metab* 93: 3478–83.

Su, H. (2010). Measuring ovarian function in young cancer survivors, *Minerva Endocrinol* 35(4): 259–70 (review).

Swain, S., Jeong, J. & Wolmark, N. (2010). Amenorrhea from breast cancer therapy – not a matter of dose, *N Engl J Med* 363(23): 2268–70.

Tanay, N. & Fenton, A. (2010). Can we predict the age of menopause transition?, *Climacteric* 13(6): 507–8.

Tham, Y., Sixton, K., Weiss, H., Elledge, R., Friedman, L. & Krame, R. (2007). The rates of chemotherapy-induced amenorrhea in patients treatd with adjuvant doxorubicin and cyclophosphamide followed by taxane, *Am. J. Clin. Oncol* 30: 126–132.

Valagussa, P., Moliterni, A., Zambetti, M. & Bonadonna, G. (1993). Long-term sequelae from adjuvant chemotherapy: recent results, *Cancer Res* 127: 247–255.

Vanhuyse, M., Fournier, C. & Bonneterre, J. (2005). Chemotherapy-induced amenorrhea influence on disease-free survival and overall survival in receptor-positive premenopausal early breast cancer patients, *Ann Oncol* pp. 1283–1288.

Vegetti, W., Marozzi, A., Manfredini, E., Testa, G., Alagna, F., Nicolosi, A., Caliari, L., Taborelli, M., Tibiletti, M., Dalpra, L. & Crosignani, P. (2000). Premature ovarian failure, *Mol Cell Endocrinol* 161: 53–57.

Walshe, J., Denduluri, N. & Swain, S. (2006). Amenorrhea in premenopausal women after chemotherapy, *J Clin Oncol* 24: 5769–5779.

Warne, G., Feirley, K., Hobbs, J. & Martin, F. (1973). Cyclophosphamide-induced ovarian failure, *New Engl J Med* 289: 1159–1162.

Welt, C., Jimenez, Y., Sluss, P., Smith, P. & Hall, J. (2006). Control of estradiol secretion in reproductive aging., *Hum Reprod* 21(8): 2189–93.

Yang, Y., Hur, N., Kim, S. & Yong, K. (2011). Correlation between sonographic and endocrine markers of ovarian aging as predictors for late menopausal transition, *Menopause* 18: 238–45.

Yu, B., Douglas, N., Ferin, M., Nakhuda, G., Crew, K., Lobo, R. & Hershman, D. (2010). Changes in markers of ovarian reserve and endocrine function in young women with breast cancer undergoing adjuvant chemotherapy, *Cancer* 116(9): 2099–105.

3

Bone Mass in Anorexia Nervosa and Thin Postmenopausal Women-Related Secondary Amenorrhea

Mário Rui Mascarenhas[1-3], Ana Paula Barbosa[1-3], Zulmira Jorge[3], Ema Nobre[3], Ana Gonçalves[3], António Gouveia de Oliveira[4] and Isabel do Carmo[3]
[1]*Endocrine Metabolism University Clinic (FMUL)*
[2]*CEDML - Endocrinology, Diabetes and Metabolism Clinic, Lda.*
[3]*Endocrinology, Diabetes and Metabolism Department*
Santa Maria Hospital, CHLN-EPE
[4]*Biostatistics Department, FCMUNL, Lisbon*
Portugal

1. Introduction

Adolescence is a critical period because there are changes in both mental and physical conditions leading to adulthood. The consequence of acute or chronic deficiency of bone mineral accumulation during adolescence may lead to severe morbidity or precocious mortality (Loro et al., 2000; Bachrach, 2001; Steelman & Zeitler, 2001)

1.1 Bone mass acquisition in normal teenagers

The first three years of life seem to be very important in the skeleton bone mass apposition. The bone mineral density (BMD) increases during childhood, but the maximum increment occurs in the critical phase of growth, reaching a plateau at the end or after the puberty in girls as well as in boys (Theintz et al., 1992; Bachrach, 2001; Schoenau et al., 2001). Bone mass increases as the bone size increase. In females, BMD is increased rapidly after 11 years of age and reaches maximum at around the age of 13-14 years or quickly after menarche. Until the age of 18 years, about 90% of the peak bone mass has been acquired. At puberty, there is an acceleration of bone mineralization, especially of the trabecular bone and by the end of sex maturation it is more than twice as compared with that at the pubertal onset (Theintz et al., 1992; Bailey, 1999).
In general, the girls have a greater BMD than boys in the first half of the second decade of life. During the intermediate stage of puberty (Martin et al., 1997), the bone mineral content (BMC) and the bone thickness are lower in girls, thus predisposing women to a higher complication risk of reduced BMD (Baroncelli & Saggese, 2000). Nutrition, body weight and total body lean mass are determinants of the bone mass in adolescent girls. Calcium intake is essential for optimization of the bone mass acquisition in healthy pubertal adolescents (Garcia e Costa et al., 1995). The accumulation of calcium in the skeleton varies with the daily intake and 1200

mg of calcium is often recommended during adolescence (Theintz et al., 1992; Ilich et al., 1997; Moreira-Andrés et al., 1995). The body weight may determine the BMD in adolescents (Cheng et al., 1998). Physical activity is known to increase the axial bone mass at the puberty (Theintz et al., 1992; Ilich et al., 1997; Bailey, 1999; Moreira-Andrés et al., 1995)

The blood levels of the thyroid hormone, growth hormone (GH), sex steroids and IGFs, which are essentially important for the skeletal growth and development, are increased during puberty. Estrogens as aromatized in osteoblasts, stimulate the GH-IGF-1 axis and may decrease bone resorption by influencing the production and activation of TGF-β and reducing the IL-6 synthesis in the bone marrow stromal cells. (Kusec et al., 1998).

2. Body composition in anorexia nervosa

Manipulations of the diet may affect the bone development during puberty. A balanced nutrition and adequate calcium intake are essential for optimal bone growth and development (Martin et al., 1997). The prevalence of anorexia nervosa is increasing in several countries of the world including in Portugal (do Carmo et al., 1996a; do Carmo et al., 2001).

The endocrine dysfunction associated with anorexia nervosa and other eating disorders may involve multiple systems and mechanisms designed to preserve energy and protect essential organs. The most affected systems are the reproductive and skeletal.

The changes in neuroendocrine signals sensitive to satiety and food intake are essentially important to keep the balance between energy store and energy expenditure. These adaptive changes include the thyroid hormone, GH, and cortisol axes, as well as the gastrointestinal tract (do Carmo et al., 1996b; Warren, 2011).

The effects of exercise on BMD are complex and incompletely understood. In premenopausal women, the changes in BMD at the proximal femur and lumbar spine differ depending on the physical activity program. Physical exercise –related beneficial effects on the BMD may be lost in intensive exercise and subsequently results in a significant loss of bone mass. Weight loss, amenorrhea, anovulation and inadequate luteal phase are evident. The effects of amenorrhea on the BMD can be mediated through the loss of body fat mass (Robinson et al., 1995).

The loss of bone mass occurs with anorexia nervosa, hypothalamic amenorrhea and in ovarian deficiencies. Replacement of estrogen and progesterone does not seem to reverse the loss of the bone mass (Karlsson et al., 2000).

2.1 Hypoestrogenism and bone mass in anorexia nervosa

Hyperprolactinemia, excessive physical activity, intense psychological stress, malnutrition and anorexia nervosa cause functional deficiency of LHRH and subsequently leads to loss of bone mass (Hergenroeder et al., 1991). Decreased pulse amplitude and frequency in the early follicular phase cause a failure of folliculogenesis and the resulting deficiency of ovarian steroids subsequently leads to loss of the bone mass (Warren, 2011). Estrogen deficiency was proposed as the main factor contributing to low BMD in anorexia nervosa.

Moreover, the degree of the BMD has been shown to be related to the duration of amenorrhea (Bachrach et al., 1991; do Carmo et al., 1994). The BMD at the lumbar spine determined by various methods is reduced in adolescent girls with amenorrhea, as compared with those who have regular cycles. However, the significant difference in BMD is found to be reversed after body weight correction (Hergenroeder et al., 1991; Karlsson et al., 2000). In fact, the increase in BMD may precede the resumption of menses in anorexic patients (Bachrach et al., 1991).

Estrogen deficiency in anorexia nervosa is an important risk factor associated with the loss of bone mass and development of osteoporosis, while malnutrition, thinness and lack of IGF-1 increase the risk of osteoporosis by estrogen-dependent and independent mechanisms (Grinspoon et al., 1999; Karlsson et al., 2000).

2.2 Other hormonal factors

In eating disorders with weight loss and poor calcium intake/absorption, the loss of bone mass is closely correlated not only with the hypoestrogenism but also with the hypercortisolism and reduced levels of IGF-1. Hypercortisolism may exacerbate hypogonadism by inhibiting GH-IGF-1 axis, reduced bone formation and increased bone resorption thus contributing to the development of osteoporosis in young patients with anorexia nervosa (Hergenroeder et al., 1991; Steelman & Zeitler, 2001).

3. Effects of anorexia nervosa on the bone mass

Understanding of the modulating factors of the BMD during adolescence is essentially important.

3.1 Adolescence

Low bone mass, which frequently causes complication in anorexic adolescent girls, occurs in the critical stage of bone development. (Kooh et al., 1996; Bachrach et al., 1991). Anorexia nervosa in adolescents may influence the linear growth and the height of the individual. The results of a study have shown that patients with anorexia nervosa had an average height of 3 cm less than the expected mean height. Reduced plasma concentration of IGF-1 may be one of the potential factors leading to reduced stature of the patients (Soyka et al., 1999). Malnutrition-associated IGF-1 deficiency may also contribute to severity of low bone mass in this population as compared to other situations of estrogen deficiency (Bachrach et al., 1991; Grinspoon et al., 1999).

Malnutrition
Intensive exercise
Calcium and Vitamin D deficiencies
Hypogonadism - hypoestrogenism
Hypercortisolism
Low IGF-1
Reduced bone formation
Increased bone resorption

Table 1. Risk factors casing reduced bone mass in the patients with anorexia nervosa.

The impact of an increased level cortisol on BMD, decreased intake of calcium and vitamin D or excessive exercise is less understood (Carmichael et al., 1995).

Intensive physical activity, especially the load-bearing exercise, has positive effects on BMD of children and adolescents. Strenuous physical activity, however delayed sexual maturation and reduced BMD (Grinspoon et al., 1999). Anorexic girls with intense physical activity also experience weight loss and amenorrhea. A study failed to demonstrate the relationship between the amount of both physical activity and BMD in normal teenage anorexic girls (Soyka et al., 1999). Some patients may have a relatively normal BMD, despite low weight, due to prior exposure to environmental (eg, pre-pubertal exercise) or hereditary factors, such as vitamin D receptor polymorphisms or COLIA 1 genes, which may have a protective function (Sainz J et al., 1997; Grinspoon et al., 1999; Sainz J et al., 1999). A study in adolescents with anorexia nervosa has shown an association between BMI and BMD (Bachrach et al., 1990). Another study has detected a marked reduction in total body fat and lean mass in girls with anorexia nervosa. However, the total lean body mass was the only variable in body composition that influenced significantly the total and regional bone. BMC at the lumbar spine and BMD at the lateral lumbar spine were detected (Soyka et al., 1999).

The severity in the degree of BMD reduction was demonstrated even in young adolescents with a short duration of this clinical condition. A marked osteopenia (or low BMD) was detected in trabecular as well as in cortical bone. The lumbar spine T-score was often 2 SD below the mean in 50% of women with anorexia nervosa (Bachrach et al., 1991).

The degree of low BMD may be enough to cause clinical fractures in several skeletal sites of women in the third decade of life and increased the risk of fragility fractures (Brotman & Stern, 1985).

The patients with amenorrhea may have marked increase in BMD during the third decade of life, which is associated with a gain in body weight and a rise in caloric intake (Karlsson et al., 2000). Girls and women with anorexia nervosa need to be rehabilitated very early in order to maximize the increase of the BMD. Early intervention is absolutely necessary. The vertebral BMD may be reduced one year after diagnosing anorexia nervosa. It was demonstrated that the women who developed anorexia nervosa before the age of 18 years, their mean BMD at the lumbar spine was found to be lower than in girls who developed anorexia nervosa later on, regardless the duration of the amenorrhea (Bachrach et al., 1991). The sexual and skeletal maturation stages were evaluated in association with the determinations of BMD: the BMD was found to be more related to stages of puberty and bone age than with the chronological age (Rubin et al., 1993).

A reduced bone mass was also found in young anorexics. (Resch H et al., 2000). Another study demonstrated bone fragility due to small size of bones originated by malnutrition and decreased volumetric BMD caused by hypoestrogenism (Karlsson et al., 2000).

The results of a research profile of the lateral lumbar spine BMD have demonstrated a marked osteopenia with a mean T-score < -1.0 SD in 63% of the cases and more than -2.0 SD in 26% of girls with anorexia nervosa (Soyka et al., 1999). A mean trabecular bone loss of 3% per year was detected in 10 adolescent girls with anorexia nervosa and amenorrhea. The onset of anorexia nervosa before acquiring the peak bone mass, and also a long-term amenorrhea may aggravate osteopenia (Bachrach et al., 1991).

Since the exact beginning of the nutritional restriction by the patient is difficult to establish, the period of disease is roughly associated with the duration of secondary amenorrhea.

Our group has evaluated the prevalence of low BMD, osteoporosis and the body soft tissues composition in Portuguese adolescent females with anorexia nervosa (Mascarenhas M et al., 2008). A subgroup of 39 adolescent girls with anorexia nervosa aged 18.6 years and mean BMI: 15.1 kg/m^2] was compared to a control subgroup of young girls and normal adult women with regular menstrual cycles [mean age: 18.9 years and mean BMI: 20.6 kg/m^2]. The BMD at the lumbar spine, at the femoral neck, at other parts of the body and the total lean and fat body masses were accessed by DXA (dual X-ray absorptiometry) using the QDR Discovery W (Hologic Inc.).

The BMI and the total fat and lean body masses were reduced in the anorexia nervosa group (P<0.0000) as well as the Also reduction in BMD at the lumbar spine, at the femoral neck, at the distal forearm and at other parts of the body was evident (Table 2). Although most of the skeleton was affected, the mean BMD was approximately 14% less in trabecular bone (measured by DXA at the lumbar spine) as compared to the control group. Our findings are consistent with the results of other study (Mascarenhas M et al., 2008).

BMD g/cm²	**ANOREXIA NERVOSA** *Age < 18 years* **Mean (±SD)**	**CONTROL SUBGROUP** *Age < 18 years* **Mean (±SD)**	***P***
L_1 - L_4	**0.856** (±0.1)	**0.992** (±0.1)	0.0167
Hip	**0.724** (±0.1)	**0.859** (±0.1)	0.0082
Distal foream	**0.518** (±0.0)	**0.555** (±0.1)	0.0432
Whole body	**1.056** (±0.1)	**1.095** (±0.1)	0.0156

BMD = bone mineral density; NSD = non-significant difference; SD = standard deviation

Table 2. The mean BMD at the lumbar spine, at the hip, at the distal forearm and at other parts of the body in the anorexia nervosa and control subgroups (adolescent girls less than 18 years old).

The portuguese adolescents with anorexia nervosa less than 18 years old had low mean total body fat and lean masses and low mean fat body percentage, as compared with the control group as seen in Table 3 (Mascarenhas M et al., 2008). Similar differences were observed by Soyka et al in 1999. In contrast to a study of Bachrach LK et al, 1991, we did not detect a reduced BMD in adolescent girls with a short duration of anorexia nervosa, Table 4 (Mascarenhas M et al., 2008). Soyka et al. (1999) found lower trabecular BMD in the lateral view of the lumbar spine. In this study the BMD at other regions of the skeleton, particularly in the proximal femur and distal forearm, were not evaluated.

	ANOREXIA NERVOSA *Age < 18 years* **Mean (±SD)**	**CONTROL SUBGROUP** *Age < 18 years* **Mean (±SD)**	***P***
Age *years*	**15.5** (±0.9)	**15.8** (±1.0)	*NSD*
Weight *kg*	**37.9** (±3.2)	**53.2** (±7.5)	*0.0000*
Height *cm*	**159.3** (±0.0)	**160.9** (±0.1)	*NSD*
BMI *kg/cm²*	**15.0** (±1.3)	**20.5** (±2.0)	*0.0000*
Total fat mass *kg*	**6.6** (±2.3)	**15.9** (±4.1)	*0.0000*
Total lean mass *kg*	**30.7** (±2.3)	**36.4** (±5.1)	*0.0000*

BMI = body mass index; NSD = non-significant difference between the means; SD = standard deviation

Table 3. The mean age, weight, height, BMI, total body fat and lean masses in between anorexia nervosa and control subgroups (girls less than 18 years old).

After adjusting the age, height and weight we did not find any contributions of the total body fat and lean masses on the BMD at the different skeletal sites in the adolescent girls with or without anorexia nervosa (Table 4). Our data differ with other studies regarding to the total lean body mass of the normal teenager group (Soyka et al., 1999; Ellis et al., 1997).

The impact of severe anorexia nervosa in the final apposition of the BMD is independent of the duration of amenorrhea and appears in females that develop the disease before 18 years old (Biller et al., 1991).

BMD g/cm^2	**ANOREXIA NERVOSA** *Age < 18 years* **Mean (±SD)**	**CONTROL SUBGROUP** *Age < 18 years* **Mean (±SD)**	***P***
L_1 - L_4	**0.846** (±0.1)	**0.925** (±0.1)	*DNS*
Hip	**0.735** (±0.1)	**0.807** (±0.1)	*DNS*
Distal foream	**0. 504** (±0.0)	**0. 515** (±0.1)	*DNS*
Whole body	**1. 049** (±0.1)	**1. 054** (±0.1)	*DNS*

BMD = bone mineral density; NSD = non-significant difference between the means; SD = standard deviation

Table 4. The mean BMD at the lumbar spine, at the hip, at the distal forearm and at other parts of the body in anorexia nervosa and control subgroups (adolescent girls less than 18 years old).

Soyka and colleagues detected that total lean body mass predicted significantly the bone mass in normal adolescent girls, but not in the anorexia nervosa group (Soyka et al., 1999). The anorexia nervosa group aged more than 18 years had also a low BMI and reduced total body fat and lean mass (Table 5). In this subgroup, the BMD at the lumbar spine, at the hip, at the distal forearm and at the other body bones were reduced, as compared to the

	ANOREXIA NERVOSA *Age < 18 years* **Mean (±SD)**	**CONTROL SUBGROUP** *Age < 18 years* **Mean (±SD)**	***P***
Age *years*	**21.0** (±3.2)	**21.0** (±3.3)	*DNS*
Weight *kg*	**40.1** (±3.9)	**55.4** (±5.9)	*0.0000*
Height *cm*	**162.1** (±0.1)	**163.3** (±0.1)	*DNS*
BMI *kg/cm^2*	**15.2** (±1.3)	**20.7** (±1.1)	*0.0000*
Total fat mass *kg*	**7.0** (±3.0)	**16.4** (±4.8)	*0.0000*
Total lean mass *kg*	**32.7** (±3.8)	**38.6** (±5.0)	*0.0000*

BMI = body mass index; NSD = non-significant difference between the means; SD = standard deviation

Table 5. The mean age, weight, height, BMI, total body fat and lean mass in anorexia nervosa and control subgroups (girls aged ≥ 18 years).

respective control subgroup (Table 6), which suggests that this group may have a greater tendency for the development of low BMD or osteoporosis in early adulthood. Grinspoon and others similarly reported that the BMD at the lumbar spine measured by DXA in 23 patients with anorexia nervosa (mean age 23 years) also reduced (Grinspoon et al., 1995). Other investigators also detected reduction of trabecular BMD at the lumbar spine (Bachrach et al., 1991; Klibanski et al., 1995; Karlsson et al., 2000).

This group of patients had a longer duration of amenorrhea, about 2 years on average, and might have a stronger negative effect on the BMD. Low bone mass in anorexia nervosa-related amenorrhea has been reported (Hergenroeder et al., 1991; Bachrach et al., 1991) However, comparison of height, weight, BMI, total body fat, lean mass and BMD measured at various skeletal regions did not show any significant difference between the anorexic subgroups under 18 years old and in patients of more than 18 years old.

In conclusion, it looks like that at an early age (up to 18 years old) there is no difference in BMD of adolescent girls with anorexia nervosa as compared with the normal. However, after the age of 18 years, there is a difference in the mean BMD between the group of patients with anorexia nervosa and the normal group, suggesting that after the age of 18 the amount of bone mineralization is more pronounced which acts as an important predictive factor for the future bone strength.

The duration of anorexic state is one of the most important predictors of reduced BMD at the lumbar spine (Soyka et al., 1999).

Our group carried out a follow-up in 15 patients with anorexia nervosa who attended the Eating Disorders Department of the Hospital de Santa Maria. The average follow-up period was of 7.6 years. The most important variable with negative correlations to bone mass recovery was disease duration (do Carmo et al, 2007). A positive correlation between bone mass recovery and the return of regular menstrual cycle was evident. However, in anorexic patients when body weight improved and menstrual cycles became regular, severe damage to bone structure was still likely to be maintained (do Carmo et al, 2007).

BMD g/cm^2	**ANOREXIA NERVOSA** *Age < 18 years* **Mean (±SD)**	**CONTROL SUBGROUP** *Age < 18 years* **Mean (±SD)**	***P***
L_1 - L_4	**0. 864** (±0.1)	**1.039** (±0.1)	*0.0014*
Hip	**0. 716** (±0.1)	**0. 894** (±0.1)	*0.0028*
Distal foream	**0. 531** (±0.0)	**0. 581** (±0.0)	*0.0098*
Whole body	**1. 061** (±0.1)	**1. 124** (±0.1)	*0.0020*

BMD = bone mineral density; NSD = non-significant difference between the means; SD = standard deviation

Table 6. The mean BMD at the lumbar spine, at the hip, at the distal forearm and at different bones of the body between anorexia nervosa and control subgroups (girls aged ≥ 18 years).

When compared, the mean BMD of 19 girls with anorexia nervosa was found to be similar to the mean BMD of 70 – 80-year-old postmenopausal women (Biller et al., 1991).

Finally, a histomorphometric study of 4 anorexic patients with low body weight showed that estrogen therapy had a very limited benefit in improving BMD and bone mass apposition (Kreipe et al., 1993).
Therefore, the severe impacts of anorexia nervosa in teenagers include retardation of linear growth, decreased bone dimension and reduced stature in adulthood (Soyka et al., 1999; Karlsson et al., 2000).

3.2 Adulthood

In 18 anorexic women (mean age: 25 years, ranging from 19 to 36 years) with amenorrhea for at least one year, a lower BMD was detected as compared with the BMD of control group. It was moreover recorded that physically inactive anorexic women had a lower BMD compared with the physically active group, suggesting that physical activity may have a protective effect (Rigotti et al., 1991).
Other studies have detected bone mass loss in the majority of women with anorexia nervosa and in 50% of those women the Z-score was 2.0 SD below the mean BMD; although both cortical and trabecular bone tissues are affected, the loss of trabecular bone is found to be more severe (Bachrach et al., 1991).
In adult women with anorexia nervosa, the mean spinal BMD had decreased about 32%, while distal radius BMD was reduced to about 18%, as compared with the control group (Bachrach et al., 1991).

4. Bone metabolism

Studies in adults with anorexia nervosa have detected a severe imbalance in bone turnover with a decrease in bone formation and an increase in bone resorption (Grinspoon et al., 1999). However, the data obtained in the adult anorexic women cannot be extrapolated to the anorexic adolescents where the rate of bone growth and mineral apposition remains active.
Bone metabolism is understudied and not fully understood in this adolescent population (Abrams et al., 1993). Most studies in adolescents with anorexia nervosa have included a small number of patients and without specific information about the markers of bone turnover, including simultaneous measurements of the bone formation/resorption markers. Other studies have included subjects with a broad age spectrum, which is from the early adolescence until early adulthood. However, the bone mass was not measured through the stages of puberty. BMD is more related to the stages of sex maturation and the bone age than the chronological age (Rubin et al., 1993).
Nutrition or calcium supplementation is directly associated with BMD, however, its impact depends on the stages of puberty (Rubin et al., 1993)
Abrams and colleagues conversely found that an increased intake of isolated calcium did not raise the BMD of adolescent girls with anorexia nervosa due to a decrease in calcium absorption with a corresponding increase in calcium excretion (Abrams et al., 1993). However, the bone markers were not evaluated in this study.
Malnutrition is associated with calcium and vitamin D deficiency (Soyka et al., 1999; Martin et al., 1997).
Saggese and colleagues demonstrated that there were changes in markers of bone formation in six adolescent patients (aged 11 to 21 years) with anorexia nervosa, but they

did not investigate other bone formation or resorption markers in these patients (Saggese et al., 1992).

The reduction of bone formation markers in anorexia nervosa is consistent with the proposed hypothesis that severe malnutrition may have a pronounced deleterious effect on functioning of the osteoblasts (Table 1). An increase in markers of bone resorption may represent increased osteoclast activity (Hotta et al., 1998; Grinspoon et al., 1999).

The biochemical markers of bone formation (osteocalcin and bone-specific alkaline phosphatase) were significantly reduced in 19 girls with anorexia nervosa. Most of the variation of bone formation in anorexia nervosa was due to the levels of IGF-1, which was found to be reduced in young women with anorexia nervosa (Soyka et al., 1999). The IGF-1 acts as an osteotrophic hormone, which affects bone growth and bone turnover by stimulating osteoblasts, collagen synthesis and longitudinal bone growth. Thus, a reduction of IGF-1 during the critical period of bone mineralization at puberty may be an important factor in the development of a low BMD in adolescents with anorexia nervosa.

The low IGF-1 plasma concentration in anorexia nervosa is correlated with reduced BMI. Therefore, IGF-1 deficicency associated with malnutrition may substantially contributes to the decrease in bone formation in the adolescents with anorexia nervosa (Golden et al., 1997; Grinspoon et al., 1999).

IGF binding proteins 2 and 3 (IGF-BP2 and IGF-BP3) plasma concentrations, the indicators of nutritional status of the individual are modified in anorexia nervosa. IGF-BP2 is increased where as IGF-BP3 is decreased in association with reduced IGF-1 as compared with the normal subjects. Moreover, the BMI correlates positively with the free IGF-1 and negatively with the IGF-BP2 (Argente et al., 1997).

Hotta and others have performed a study in Japanese anorexic youth submitted to intravenous nutrition. The results revealed that the improvement of nutritional status was associated with rapid and marked increase in plasma levels of osteocalcin and IGF-1 (Hotta et al., 1998).

5. Bone mass during the recovery of anorexia nervosa

Therapeutic strategies to stimulate bone mass recovery in patients with anorexia nervosa need to be carefully formulated. A study conducted in New York showed that just a mean weight of approximately 90% of the desirable body weight, spontaneous menses return in 86% of patients within the next 6 months (Golden et al., 1997). Therefore, 90% of desirable weight seems to be a reasonable target for weight gain therapy. Resumption of menses was obviously associated with the activation of the hypothalamic-pituitary-ovarian axis (also associated with total body fat mass). It was concluded that plasma levels of 17β-estradiol is the best marker for determining the resumption of menstrual cycle (Golden et al., 1997).

Studies conducted up to 8 years after the onset of anorexia nervosa showed that only 48% of patients recovered normal body weight and showed regular menstrual cycles (Herzog et al., 1993).

However, the BMD at the lumber spine of 69 women at various stages of recovery from anorexia nervosa showed a decrease in BMD compared to controls. Even exercise did not show any protective effect on the skeleton in these patients. BMD in these women was moreover associated with the duration of amenorrhea (Hay et al., in 1992).

A group of 51 women with anorexia nervosa was investigated during 11.7 years. In these patients measurements of BMD were made at the lumbar spine and forearm. Groups were divided into three according to their stages of recovery:

a. a good recovery - women who had regular cycles and not weighed less than 85% of their expected body weight,
b. a poor recovery - the patients who had not reached regular cycles and weighed less than 85%,
c. an intermediate stage of recovery - the patients had not yet achieved regular cycles but their body weight was found to be higher than 85% of expected body weight.

The group of patients with good recovery had a significantly increased BMD at the lumbar spine and at the forearm as compared with the other two groups. The group with an intermediate recovery type had a higher BMD at the lumbar spine than the group with a poor recovery. It was concluded from this study that the recovery of trabecular bone mass is achieved by a successful treatment of anorexia, but the recovery of cortical bone mass is comparatively slow and gradual. (Herzog et al., 1993).

Independent effect of weight gain in improving BMD and in the absence of estrogen therapy have also been reported(Bachrach et al., 1991; Rigotti et al., 1991; Herzog et al., 1993).

A Canadian study in Toronto showed that bone mass was strongly correlated with lean tissue in anorexia nervosa while its relation with the body fat mass was weaker. However, the follow-up of anorexic patients for 7 to 26 months showed a modest increase in weight (average 4.9 kg), which was due primarily to an increase in body fat mass with a slight and insignificant increase in lean body mass. Bone mass remained almost unchanged or even decreased in some cases. Only 4 patients gained normal body weight (BMI > 20 kg/m^2) and had normal menstrual cycles, but the bone mass in these four responders did not increase. In this study the authors demonstrated that the adolescent girls with anorexia nervosa restore bone mass following an increment of the soft body mass/tissue. (Kooh et al., 1996).

A swiss study showed that bone mass decreased 6 to 28% despite nutritional and body weight recovery (Ruegsegger et al., 1988).

According to Hotta and colleagues, an increase in BMD and normalization of bone formation and resorption markers occur if the BMI is above 16.5 kg/m^2. The yearly BMD increment is BMI dependent in young patients recovering from anorexia nervosa (Hotta et al., 1998). The retrospective data of Valla and his colleagues showed a recovery of BMD in those who regained body weight and regular menstrual cycles and suggested that in addition to body weight other factors, such as menstrual disorders and hypoestrogenism are independent and additive risk factors causing loss of bone mass in patients with anorexia nervosa (Valla et al., 2000).

In hypoestrogenism, the impact of hormone therapy on bone mass depends on pathogenesis, hormone administration route and the dosage used (Bruni et al., 2000).

A survey of Robinson and his colleagues revealed that most of the clinicians dealing with anorexia nervosa prescribe contraceptive pills for the treatment of low BMD despite its poor effectiveness in preventing or reversing anorexia-associated conditions (Karlsson et al., 2000; Kreipe et al., 1993; Bruni et al., 2000).

Klibanski et al. studied 48 women with anorexia nervosa (mean age 23.7 years old) and reported that the BMD at the lumbar spine did not change after 1.5 years of estrogen therapy. However, about 4% increase in BMD was evident in the treated patients who had less than 70% of the desirable body weight. In contrast, in women not receiving estrogen therapy, the BMD decreased by 20%. The patients who regained spontaneous menstrual cycles had a 19.3% increase in bone mass (Klibanski et al., 1995). Other authors, however, found that the oral contraceptives used in anorexia nervosa were associated with an increased BMD all over the body including at the lumbar spine (Seeman et al, 1992).

6. Bone complications in anorexia nervosa

The persistent low bone mass often a common complication of anorexia nervosa in the adolescent population may cause increased risk of spontaneous and/or clinical fractures (Kooh et al., 1996 ; Bachrach et al., 1991; Brotman & Stern, 1985; Herzog et al., 1993).

The degree of reduced bone mass may cause severe complications. Women with anorexia nervosa and one year of amenorrhea had multiple crash vertebral fractures (Rigotti et al., 1991).

A study revealed collapse of the femoral head in a short stature 20 year-old anorexic dancer. This patient had delayed bone age (13 years), primary amenorrhea and hypoestrogenism. The possible osteonecrosis mechanisms included repeated micro-traumas (Warren et al., 1990).

However, a study performed by Hartman and colleagues in 19 women who recovered from anorexia nervosa for more than 20 years showed that recovery from clinical disease did not confer a normal bone mass (Hartman et al., 2000).

Marked osteoporosis can develop in young adult women with persistent amenorrhea and anorexia nervosa. Unlike other forms of pre-menopausal osteoporosis, fractures in these patients at the various regions of the skeleton are common, with a 7-fold increased risk for nonvertebral fractures as compared with women of the same age (Steelman & Zeitler, 2001; Heaney R., 1998; Rigotti et al., 1991).

7. Thin postmenopausal women

Aging in both sexes is accompanied by loss of muscle mass and strength. Muscle weakness may harm the quality of life and autonomy of elderly people.

The decline of lean body mass that occurs with aging probably includes a decrease in somatotropin (GH) synthesis and secretion due to decreased pituitary response to GHRH, loss of muscle fibers, neuromuscular changes, sedentary lifestyle and other changes intrinsically associated with aging (Douchi et al., 1998).

In the pre-menopausal women, the response to GHRH is increased which is not found in the post-menopausal women, suggesting that the age-related decline in GH results in the loss of muscle mass (Douchi et al., 1998). Bone loss accelerates substantially in the late perimenopause and continues at a similar pace in the first postmenopausal years (Gillette-Guyonnet et al., 2000; Finkelstein J. et al, 2008).

In the post-menopause, the lean mass of the trunk, lower limb and of the total body, measured by DXA, is lower than in the premenopausal women and is inversely related to age and menopause duration. In postmenopausal women the loss of lean body mass is independent of the age and bodyweight. The lean body mass of the trunk declines more quickly than other areas of the body (Finkelstein J. et al, 2008). Addition of androgen to estrogen therapy increases lean body mass in postmenopausal women (Davis, S., 1999).

A study of 129 women aged between 75 to 89 years showed that muscle mass was significantly reduced along with the incidence of osteoporosis and reduced BMD at the hip. It was concluded that the lean body mass has a protective effect on BMD at the femoral neck (Gillette-Guyonnet et al., 2000). So far, it is unclear whether lean mass regulates the bone mass in the postmenopausal women. The importance of lean mass or muscle mass in controlling the bone mass is supported by in vitro and in vivo studies. The results of autopsies after adjusting body weight, age and height showed that there was a significant relation between the weight of the ashes of the third vertebra of the spine and the left psoas weight; another investigation revealed the existence of a correlation between the lumbar spine extensor muscles strength and BMD at the lumbar spine (Aloia et al., 1991). A study in women of more than 60 years old revealed that the lean body mass contributed significantly to predict the cancellous BMD (Aloia et al., 1991). However, no correlation between the whole body potassium and the BMD at the trochanter or Ward's triangle was evident (Aloia et al., 1991). The duration of fertility period but not the age at menarche or at menopause may affect osteoporosis?. The obstetric history of previous childbirths and/or miscarriages, independent of the number, is not a risk factor for osteopenia or osteoporosis?

8. Contribution of lean and fat mass to bone mass

The body fat tends to increase with age. Most of the studies match the importantance of the body weight in determining the BMD, especially in the axial skeleton. However, the relative contribution of both the lean and fat body masses in BMD is not evident. In the transition to menopause, the BMI and the total body fat mass are increased. Also the lean body mass and bone mass are decreased, while the fat mass increases in postmenopausal women (android distribution). It however, remains unclear whether the changes are due to age or to menopause (Tremollieres et al., 1996; Douchi et al., 1998; Ijuin H et al., 1999; Wang Q et al., 1994).

A longitudinal study showed that a rapid increase in visceral fat mass generally attributed to the aging process (Tchernof et al., 1998). Moreover, a total body fat mass assessed by DXA in postmenopausal women could predict BMD at the spine and at the hip.

The decreased fat mass is a risk factor for osteoporotic fractures, because 11% to 15% of patients with fragility fractures showed low fat mass, whereas the lean body mass in the same patients remained the same compared to controls; in women aged more than 75 years, a protective effect of body weight and fat mass on BMD at several skeletal sites was positively correlated with the weight and the fat mass (Gillette-Guyonnet et al., 2000).

A swedish study, on the other hand, compared urban and rural populations and found that the incidence of osteoporotic fractures was higher only in a group of women more than 70 years old with reduced muscle mass, which highlighted the importance of the muscle mass as a primary agent influencing the bone mass changes and the fracture risk in elderly women (Elmstahl et al., 1993).

We have evaluated a group of 53 thin postmenopausal women (BMI < 18.5 kg/m^2). The BMD measurements at the lumbar spine, at the femoral neck and at other parts of the body and the total lean and fat body masses were also accessed. The Z-scores and the T-scores were also determined. Our results revealed that in the post-menopausal patients, osteoporosis was associated with low BMI. The mean Z-scores of the BMD were at the lumbar spine -1.1 SD, at the femoral neck -1.2 SD and at the total hip -1.3 SD, respectively (Mascarenhas M et al., 2003). These data may suggest that low body weight and reduced

BMI in the postmenopausal women may also exacerbate the loss of bone mass as well as enhance the development of osteoporosis. The results are also consistent with the previous data presented on the protective effects of both the total fat mass and body weight on BMD. (Mascarenhas M et al., 2003; Mascarenhas M et al., 2004).
A study in postmenopausal Chinese women with type 2 diabetes mellitus (T2DM) showed a higher osteoporosis risk for the hipbone compared to the lumbar spine, especially in those with a BMI below 18kg/m^2. (Peng-Fei S et al, 2009).

9. Conclusion

In anorexia nervosa and control adolescent women, the mean BMD were similar, but the BMD at the femoral neck and at the lumbar spine showed a tendency to decrease between 8.5% to 9% in the anorexic patients. However, secondary amenorrhea of about 10 months duration may be short in exerting any significant difference in BMD at several skeletal sites.
The anorectic patients were found to be lighter with low total body fat and lean body mass compared to controls of the same age. In these adolescents with or without anorexia nervosa, total body fat and lean mass do not contribute to BMD at the diverse regions of the skeleton.
In the patients of anorexia nervosa aged over 18 years, the BMD at the lumbar spine, femoral neck, distal forearm and at different bone of the body were significantly reduced, suggesting that these girls may have higher tendency to develop low BMD or osteoporosis in their early adulthood. These patients also showed a longer duration of amenorrhea (about 2 years on average), which might have a greater impact on the BMD. In the anorexic patients aged more than 18 years, a positive correlation between the total body fat to the BMD at the femoral neck and at different regions of the bones were observed. The data suggest a direct link between the nutritional status and BMD in patients with anorexia nervosa.
The current consensus on the relative contribution of the total body fat and lean mass to BMD at different bones of the body in the postmenopausal patients comes from the evidence of the most cross-sectional studies.
Longitudinal studies to assess BMD in postmenopausal women are essential to know whether the changes in BMD are sensitive to changes in body composition and to delineate the mechanism involved.
Finally, it seems to be very important to know that young women with anorexia nervosa and the thin postmenopausal women should be identified in advance in order to modify their behavior and consequent reduction in the future risk of osteoporosis and the fragility fractures.

10. References

Abrams, S., Silber, T. & Esteban, N. 1993. Mineral balance and bone turnover in adolescents with anorexia nervosa. *J Pediatr* Vol. 123, 1993, pp. 326-331

Aloia, J., McGowan, D., Vaswani, A., Ross, P. & Cohn, S. 1991. Relationship of menopause to skeletal and muscle mass. *Am J Clin Nutr* Vol. 53, 1991, pp. 1378-1383

Argente, J., Caballo, N., Barrios, V., Muñoz, M., Pozo, J., Chowen, J., Morandé, G. & Hernández, M. 1997. Multiple endocrine abnormalities of the growth hormone and insulin-like growth factor axis in patients with anorexia nervosa: effect of short-

and long-term weight recuperation. *J Clin Endocrinol Metab* Vol. 82, 1997, pp. 2084-2092

Bachrach LK. 2001. Acquisition of optimal bone mass in childhood and adolescence. *Trends in Endocrinology and Metabolism* Vol. 12, 2001, pp. 22-28

Bachrach, L., Guido, D., Katzman, D., Litt, I. & Marcus, R. 1990. Decreased bone density in adolescent girls with anorexia nervosa. *Pediatrics* Vol. 86, 1990, pp. 440-447

Bachrach, L., Katzman, D., Litt, I., Guido, D. & Marcus, R. 1991a. Recovery from osteopenia in adolescent girls with anorexia nervosa. *J Clin Endocrinol Metab* Vol. 72, 1991, 602-606

Bailey DA. 1999. A six-year longitudinal study of the relationship of physical activity to bone mineral accrual in growing children: the University of Saskatchewan Bone Mineral Accrual Study. *J Bone Miner Res* Vol. 14, 1999, pp. 1672-1679

Baroncelli, G., & Saggese, G. 2000. Critical Ages and Stages of Puberty in the Accumulation of Spinal and Femoral Bone Mass: The Validity of Bone Mass Measurements. *Hormone Research* Vol. 54 (Suppl 1), 2000, pp. 2-8

Biller, B., Coughlin, J., Saxe, V., Schoenfeld, D., Spratt, D. & Klibanski, A. 1991. Osteopenia in women with hypothalamic amenorrhea: a prospective study. *Obstet Gynecol* Vol. 78, 1991, pp. 996-1001

Brotman, A. & Stern, T. 1985. Osteoporosis and pathologic fractures in anorexia nervosa. *Am J Psychiatry* Vol. 142, 1985, pp. 495-496

Bruni, V., Dei, M., Vicini, I., Beninato, L & Magnani L. 2000. Estrogen replacement therapy in the management of osteopenia related to eating disorders. *Ann N Y Acad Sci* Vol. 900, 2000, pp. 416-421

Carmichael, K., & Carmichael, D. Bone metabolism and osteopenia in eating disorders. 1995. *Medicine* Vol. 74, 1995, pp. 254-267

Cheng, J., Leung, S., Lee, W., Lau, J., Maffulli, N., Cheung, A. & Chan, K. 1998. Determinants of axial and peripheral bone mass in Chinese adolescents. *Arch Dis Child* Vol. 78, 1998, pp. 524-530

Davis SR. 1999. Androgen Replacement in Women: A Commentary. *J Clin Endocrinol Metab* Vol. 84, 1999, pp. 1886-1891

do Carmo, I., Mascarenhas, M., Macedo, A., Silva, A., Santos, I., Bouça, D., Myatt, J., & Sampaio, D. 2007. A Study of Bone Density Change in Patients with Anorexia Nervosa. *Eur Eat Disorders Ver* Vol. 15, 2007, pp. 457–462

do Carmo, I., Reis, D., Jorge, Z. & Galvão-Teles, A. 1994. Gonadotrophic function and starvation in anorexia nervosa. *Eur J Endocrinol* Vol. 130 (suppl 2), 1994, pp. 167

do Carmo, I., Reis, D., Sampaio, D. & Galvão-Teles, A. 1996b. Fonction thyroidienne, index de masse corporelle et pourcentage de perte de poids au cours de l'anorexie mentale. *Rev Franc Endocrinol Clin* Vol. 37, 1996, pp. 489-494

do Carmo, I., Reis, D., Varandas, P., Bouça, D., Padre-Santo, D., Neves, A., André, I., Sampaio, D. & Galvão-Teles, A. 1996a. Prevalence of anorexia nervosa: a portuguese population study. *Eur Eating Dis Rev*, Vol. 4, 1996, pp. 157-170

do Carmo, I., Reis, D., Varandas, P., Bouça, D., Padre-Santo, D., Neves, A., André, I., Sampaio, D. & Galvão-Teles, A. Epidemiologia da anorexia nervosa: prevalência da anorexia nervosa em adolescentes do sexo feminino nos distritos de Lisboa e Setúbal. 2001. *Acta Médica Portuguesa* Vol. 14, 2001, pp. 301-316

Douchi, T., Yamamoto, S., Nakamura, S., Ijuin, T., Oki, T., Maruta, K. & Nagata, Y. 1998. The effect of menopause on regional and total body lean mass. Maturitas Vol. 29, 1998, pp. 247-252

Ellis, K., Abrams, S. & Wong, W. 1997. Body composition of a young, multiethnic female population. *Am J Clin Nutr* Vol. 65, 1997, pp. 724-731

Elmstahl, S., Gardsell, P., Ringsberg, K. & Sernbo, I. 1993. Body composition and its relation to bone mass and fractures in an urban and rural population. *Aging Clin Exp Res* Vol. 5, 1993, pp. 47-54

Finkelstein, J., Brockwell, S., Mehta, V., Greendale, G., Sowers, M., Ettinger, B., Lo, J., Johnston, J., Cauley, J., Danielson, M. & Neer, R. 2008. Bone Mineral Density Changes during the Menopause Transition in a Multiethnic Cohort of Women. *J Clin Endocrinol Metab* Vol. 93, 2008, pp. 861–868

Garcia-e-Costa, J., Mascarenhas, M., Gouveia-de-Oliveira, A. & Galvão-Teles, A. 1994. Total Fat and Lean Body Masses and Bone Density Gain in Boys and Girls. *Int J Obesity* Vol. 18(Sup 2), 1994, pp. 26

Gillette-Guyonnet, S., Nourhashemi, F., Lauque, S., Grandjean, H. & Vellas B. 2000. Body Composition and osteoporosis in elderly women. *Gerontology* Vol. 46, 2000, pp. 189-193

Golden, N., Jacobson, M., Schebendach, J., Solanto, M., Hertz, S. & Shenker, I. 1997. Resumption of menses in anorexia nervosa. *Arch Pediatr Adolesc Med* Vol. 151, 1997, pp. 16-21

Grinspoon, S., Baum, H., Kim, V., Coggins, C. & Klibanski, A. 1995. Decreased bone formation and increased mineral dissolution during acute fasting in young women. *J Clin Endocrinol Metab* Vol. 80, 1995, pp. 3628-3633

Grinspoon, S., Miller, K., Coyle, C., Krempin, J., Armstrong, C., Pitts, S., Herzog, D., & Klibanski A. 1999. Severity of Osteopenia in Estrogen-Deficient Women with Anorexia Nervosa and Hypothalamic Amenorrhea. *J Clin Endocrinol Metab* Vol. 84, 1999, pp. 2049-2055

Hartman, D., Crisp, A., Rooney, B., Rackow, C., Atkinson, R. & Patel, S. 2000. Bone density of women who have recovered from anorexia nervosa. *Int J Eat Disord* Vol. 28, 2000. pp. 107-112

Hay, P., Delahunt, J., Hall, A., Mitchell, A., Harper, G. & Salmond, C. 1992. Predictors of osteopenia in premenopausal women with anorexia nervosa. *Calcif Tissue Int* Vol. 50, 1992, pp. 498-501

Heaney, R. 1998. Osteoporosis: pathophysiology of osteoporosis. *Endocrinol Metab Clin* Vol. 27, 1998, pp. 255-265

Hergenroeder, A., Fiorotto, M. & Klish W. 1991. Body composition in ballet dancers measured by total body electrical conductivity. *Med Sci Sports Exerc* Vol. 23, 1991, pp. 528-533

Herzog, W., Minne, H., Deter, C., Leidig, G., Schellberg, D. & Bluster, C. 1993. Outcome of bone mineral density in anorexia nervosa patients 11.7 years after first admission. *J Bone Miner Res* Vol. 8, 1993, pp. 597-605

Hotta, M., Shibasaki, T., Sato, K. & Demura, H. 1998. The importance of body weight history in the occurrence and recovery of osteoporosis in patients with anorexia nervosa;

evaluation by dual x-ray absorptiometry and bone metabolic markers. *Eur J Endocrinol* Vol. 139, 1998, pp. 276-283

Ijuin, H., Douchi, T., Oki, T., Maruta, K. & Nagata, Y. 1999. The contribution of menopause to changes in body-fat distribution. J Obstet Gynaecol Res Vol. 25, 1999, pp. 367-372

Ilich, J., Badenhop, N., Jelic, T., Clairmont, A., Nagode, L., & Matkovic, V. 1997. Calcitriol and bone mass accumulation in females during puberty. *Calcif Tissue Int* Vol. 61, 1997, pp. 104-109

Kaplan, F., Pertschuk, M., Fallon, M. & Haddad J. 1985. Osteoporosis and hip fracture in a young woman with anorexia nervosa. *Clin Orthop Rel Res* Vol. 212, 1985, pp. 250-254

Karlsson, M., Weigall, S., Duan Y. & Seeman E. 2000. Bone size and volumetric density in women with anorexia nervosa receiving estrogen replacement therapy and in women recovered from anorexia nervosa. *J Clin Endocrinol Metab* Vol. 85, 2000, pp. 3177-3182

Klibanski, A., Biller, B., Schoenfeld, D., Herzog, D. & Saxe, V. 1995. The effects of estrogen administration on trabecular bone loss in young women with anorexia nervosa. *J Clin Endocrinol Metabolism* Vol. 80, 1995, pp. 898-904

Kooh, S., Noriega, E., Leslie, K., Muller, C. & Harrison, J. 1996. Bone mass and soft tissue composition in adolescents with anorexia nervosa. *Bone*, Vol. 19, 1996, pp. 181-188

Kusec, V., Virdi, A., Prince R. & Triffit J. 1998. Localization of estrogen receptor-alpha in human and rabbit skeletal tissues. *J Clin Endocrinol Metab* 1998, Vol. 83, pp. 2421-2428

Loro, M., Sayre, J., Roe, T., Goran, M., Kaufman, F., & Gilsanz, V. 2000. Early Identification of Children Predisposed to Low Peak Bone Mass and Osteoporosis Later in Life. *J Clin Endocrinol Metab* Vol. 85, 2000, pp. 3908-3918

Martin, A., Bailey, D., McKay, H., & Whiting, S. 1997. Bone mineral and calcium accretion during puberty. *Am J Clin Nutr* Vol. 66, 1997, pp. 611-615

Mascarenhas, M., Guerra, S., Camolas, J., Almeida, F., Lança, V., Negreiro, F., Breitenfeld, L., Gouveia de Oliveira, A., Bicho, M., Galvão-Teles, A. 2003. Menopause Age, Post-Menopausal Years, Height and Weight: How to Predict the Osteoporosis? *Annals of the Rheumatic Diseases* Vol. 62 (Suppl. 1), 2003, pp. 321

Mascarenhas, M., Guerra, S., Camolas, J., Galvão-Teles, A., Jacinto, D., Santos Pinto, D., Bicho, M. 2004. Abdominal adipose tissue in post-menopause women with and without cardiovascular risk and with cardiovascular complications. *International Journal of Obesity and Related Metabolic Disorders* Vol. 28 (Suppl. 1), 2004, pp. S124

Mascarenhas, M., Vieira, J., Jorge, Z., Nobre, E., Camolas, J., Carvalho, M., Duarte, D. & do Carmo, I. 2008. Relações da massa magra e da massa óssea em jovens do sexo feminino com anorexia nervosa. In Abstracts Book of the 2008 SPODOM Congress. 2008, pp. 7-8

Moreira-Andrés, M., Papapietro, K., Cañizo, F., Rejas, J., Larrodera, L., Hawkins, F. 1995. Correlations between bone mineral density, insulin-like growth factor I and auxological variables. *Eur J Endocrinol* Vol. 132, 1995, pp. 573-9

Peng-Fei S., Xian-Ping W., Hong Z., Xing-Zhi C., Wei G., Xiao-Ge D., Chi G. & Er-Yuan L. 2009. Bone mineral density and its relationship with body mass index in postmenopausal women with type 2 diabetes mellitus in mainland China. *J Bone Miner Metab* 2009, vol. 27, pp. 190–197

Resch, H., Newrkla, S., Grampp, S., Resch, A., Zapf, S., Piringer, S., Hockl, A. & Weiss, P. 2000. Ultrasound and X-ray-based bone densitometry in patients with anorexia nervosa. *Calcif Tissue Int* 2000, Vol. 66, pp. 338-341

Rigotti, N., Neer, R., Skates, S., Herzog, D. & Nussbaum, S. 1991. The clinical course of osteoporosis in anorexia nervosa. *JAMA* Vol. 265, 1991. pp. 1133-1138

Robinson, T., Snow-Harter, C., Taaffe, D., Gillis, D., Shaw, J. & Marcus R. 1995. Gymnasts exhibit higher bone mass than runners despite similar prevalence of amenorrhea and oligomenorrhea. *J Bone Miner Res* Vol. 10, 1995, pp. 26-35

Rubin, K., Schirduan, V., Gendreau, P., Sarfarazi, M., Mendola, R. & Dalsky, G. 1993. Predictors of axial and peripheral bone mineral density in healthy children and adolescents, with special attention to the role of puberty. *J Pediatr* Vol. 123, 1993, pp. 863-870

Ruegsegger, P., Muller, A., Dambacher, M., Ittner, J., Willi, J. & Kopp, H. 1988. Bone loss in female patients with anorexia nervosa. Schweiz Med Wochenschr Vol. 118, 1988, 233-238

Saggese, G., Bertelloni, S., Baroncelli, G. & DiNero, G. 1992. Serum levels of carboxyterminal propeptide of type 1 procollagen in healthy children from 1st year of life to adulthood and in metabolic bone diseases. *Eur J Pediatr* Vol 151, 1992, pp. 764-820

Sainz, J., van Tornout, J, Loro, M., Sayre, J., Roe, T. & Gilsanz, V. 1997. Vitamin D receptor gene polymorphisms and bone density in prepubertal girls. *N Engl J Med* Vol. 337, 1997, pp. 77-82

Sainz, J., van Tornout, J., Sayre, J., Kaufman, F. & Gilsanz V. 1999. Association of collagen type 1 a1 gene polymorphism with bone density in early childhood. *J Clin Endocrinol Metab* Vol. 84, 1999, pp.853-855

Schoenau, E., Neu, C., Rauch, F., & Manz, F. 2001. The Development of Bone Strength at the Proximal Radius during Childhood and Adolescence. *J Clin Endocrinol Metab* Vol.86, 2001, pp. 613-618

Seeman, E., Szmukler, G.I., Formica, C., Tsalamandris, C., Mestrovic, R. 1992. Osteoporosis in anorexia nervosa: the influence of peak bone density, bone loss, oral contraceptive use, and exercise. *J Bone Miner Res*, 1992;7:1467-1474

Soyka, L., Grinspoon, S., Levitsky, L., Herzog, D. & Klibanski, A. 1999. The Effects of Anorexia Nervosa on Bone Metabolism in Female Adolescents. *J Clin Endocrinol Metab*, Vol. 84, 1999, pp. 4489-4496

Steelman J., & Zeitler, P. 2001. Osteoporosis in Pediatrics. *Pediatr Rev* Vol. 22, 2001, pp. 56-64

Tchernof, A., Poehlman, E. 1998. Effects of the menopause transition on body fatness and body fat distribution. Obes Res Vol. 6, 1998, pp. 246-254

Theintz, G., Buchs, B., Rizzoli, R., Slosman, D., Clavien, H., Sizonenko, P., & Bonjour, J. 1992. Longitudinal monitoring of bone mass accumulation in healthy adolescents: evidence for a marked reduction after 16 years of age at the levels of lumbar spine and femoral neck in female subjects. *J Clin Endocrinol Metab* Vol. 75, 1992, pp. 1060-1065

Tremollieres, F., Pouilles, J-M. & Ribot, C. 1996. Relative influence of age and menopause on total and regional body composition changes in postmenopausal women. *Am J Obstet Gynecol* Vol. 175, 1996, pp. 1594-1600

Valla, A., Groenning, I., Syversen, U. & Hoeiseth A. 2000. Anorexia nervosa: slow regain of bone mass. *Osteoporos Int* Vol. 11, 2000, pp. 141-145

Wang, Q., Hassager, C., Ravn, P., Wang, S. & Christiansen C. 1994. Total and regional body-composition changes in early postmenopausal women: age-related or menopause-related? *Am J Clin Nutr* Vol. 60, 1994, pp. 843-848

Warren, M., Shane, E., Lee, M., Lindsay, R., Dempster, D., Warren, L., Hamilton, W. 1990. Femoral head collapse associated with anorexia nervosa in a 20-year-old ballet dancer. Clin Orthop Vol. 51, 1990, pp. 171-176

Warren, P. 2011. Endocrine Manifestations of Eating Disorders. *J Clin Endocrinol Metab* Vol. 96, 2011, pp. 333-343

4

Polycystic Ovary Syndrome

Ingrid Dravecká and Ivica Lazúrová
*Department of Internal Medicine, Medical Faculty, University Košice
Slovakia*

1. Introduction

1.1 Definition

Polycystic ovary syndrome (PCOS) is a remarkably common disorder of premenopausal women with a prevalence of 5-10%. Besides reproductive endocrine abnormalities, including amenorrhea or oligomenorrhea, hyperandrogenism and infertility, patients with PCOS often show an insulin resistance and beta-cell dysfunction (1).

1.2 Diagnostic criteria

The condition was described by Stein and Leventhal in 1935. There is a considerable controversy on the optimal criteria for PCOS. Although the **NIH** (National Institute of Health) **criteria** as hyperandrogenic anovulatory PCOS were proposed in 1992, these have now expanded to **non NIH criteria** including hyperandrogenic ovulatory to non-hyperandrogenic anovulatory PCOS (2). After a meeting between ESHRE (European Society for Human Reproduction and Embryology) and ASRM (American Society for Reproductive Medicine) in Rotterdam in 2003, a new set of criteria for PCOS was proposed, commonly refered to as **Rotterdam criteria**: 1. irregular/no ovulations, 2. clinical/paraclinical hyperandrogenemia and 3. polycystic ovaries. Two out of the three criteria need to be fulfilled and other causes of hyperandrogenemia should by excluded. The Rotterdam criteria are curently debated because they introduced two new fenotypes (3). It is known that the metabolic disturbances of PCOS are more pronounced in hyperandrogen patients compared to patients with no hyperandrogenemia in genetic studies. In 2006 AES (Androgen Excess Society) published a position statement which suggested that androgen excess is the key component of PCOS related to clinical symptoms and long-term morbidity. According to **AES**, diagnostic **criteria** should be modified to include only those with hyperandrogenism and polycystic ovary or ovarian dysfunction (2). This definition excluded the phenotype subset of polycystic ovary and ovarian dysfunction without hyperandrogenism.

NIH criteria covered first two phenotypes: A and B, Rotterdam criteria covered all four phenotypes (including non hyperandrogenic anovulatory polycystic ovary) and finally AES criteria excluded non-hyperandrogenic phenotype Table 1 (2).

These criteria recognize that PCOS is a functional disorder in which ovarian hyperandrogenism can occur in the presence or absence of ovarian morphologic changes. However, according to Rotterdam criteria or AES criteria, polycystic ovaries need not to be present to make a diagnosis of PCOS and controversely their presence alone does not establish the diagnosis of PCOS (2).

Features	**Phenotypes**						
	A	B	C	D	E	F	G
Hyperandrogenism (biochemical/clinical)	+	+	+	-	+	-	-
Oligo - or anovulation	+	+	-	+	-	-	+
Polycystic ovaries	+	-	+	+	-	+	-
NIH criteria	√	√					
ESHRE/ASRM criteria	√	√	√	√			
AES criteria	√	√	√				

Table 1. Comparison of the different reproductive diagnostic criteria for PCOS resulting in potentially different phenotypes (2)

1.3 Ethiopathogenesis

Although exact pathogenic mechanisms of PCOS are still not completely rocognised, most of factors involved in the development of PCOS can be devided into following groups:

- Aberration of gonadotropic secretion
- Genetics
- Environmental factors
- Hyperinsulinemia and insulin resistance

1.4 Aberration of gonadotropic secretion

It is well known, that gonadotropin-releasing hormone (GnRH) pulse frequency is accelerated in PCOS. However, it is not clear whether this accelerated pulse frequency is primarily or secondarily to the relatively low levels of progesterone resulting in rare ovulatory events. Both situations lead to an increase luteinizing hormone (LH) levels resulting in increased ovarian androgen production (4).

1.5 Genetics

Lines of evidence suggest that PCOS is a heritable disorder. Various approaches have been undertaken to try to define a specific genetic etiology. While a number of candidate genes appear to make modest contributions to the clinical expression of PCOS, no single gene has been confidentaly identified to play a predominant role in the pathogenesis of PCOS.
Family studies showed a PCOS prevalence of 25-50% in first degree relatives of patients with PCOS, suggesting a strong inheritance of PCOS. PCOS is a heterogenous disease and the genetic profile of different phenotypes may differ (5). In the study of Franks et al. authors compared metabolic and hormonal parametres of probands with PCOS and oligoamenorrhea with affected sisters with ultrasound findings of polycystic ovary. Although affected sisters had fewer symptoms that probands, serum testosterone, LH and insulin sensitivity index were similar in both groups. Affected sisters had also the higher frequency of oligomenorrhea, hirsutism and other hyperandrogenic symptoms. Thus authors demostrated a moderate to high heritability for all traits studied in affected pairs Figure 1, Figure 2 (6).

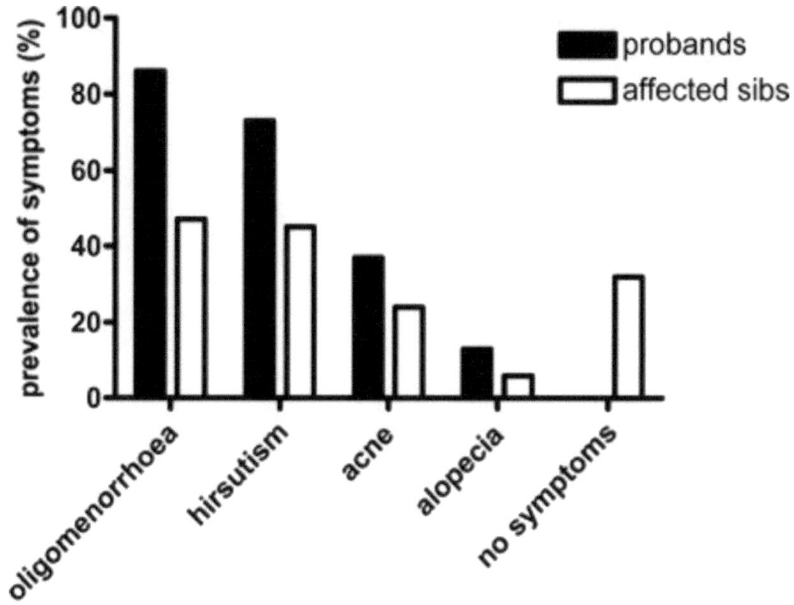

Fig. 1. Distribution of symptoms in probands with PCOS and affected sisters (6).

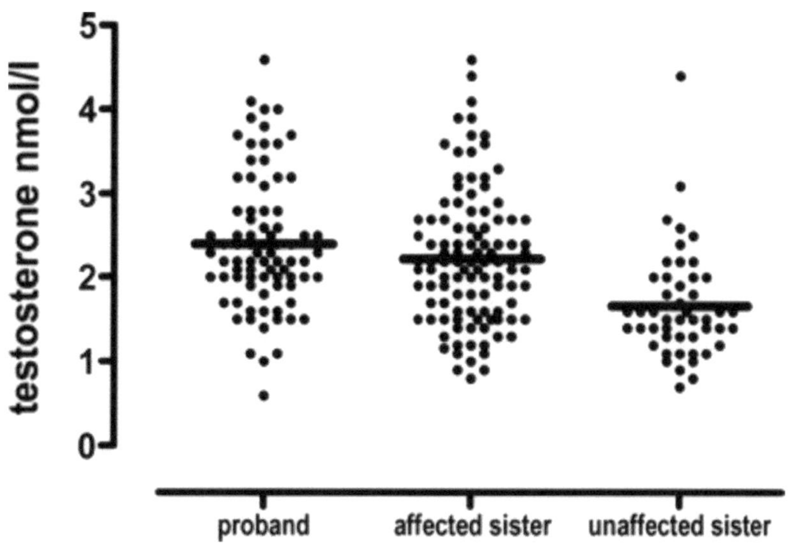

Fig. 2. Serum testosterone concentrations in individual probands, affected sisters, and unaffected sisters (6).

The most commonly used method for evaluation of the genetic profile in PCOS has been the candidate gene approach. Using this approach, severel genes involved in androgen synthesis, secretion, metabolism and regulation have been evaluated along with group of genes affecting insulin resistance, insulin secretion and inflammation. Candidate genes studies however brought only few informations. Genome wide association studies are likely to be more informative. Recent sudies therefore applied DNA microarrays to evaluate differences in gene expresion in different tissues between PCOS patients and controls. Results of these studies may be used to achieve new knowledge of the pathogenesis of PCOS which is still unknown. Like other common dissease such as diabetes mellitus type 2, PCOS is most likely a multigenetic dissease with several genes having small and additive effect.

Locus on chromosome 19p13 2 appears to be most promissing candidate gene locus. Genes involved in the serin phosphorylation of the insulin receptor (INS VNTR, CYP 11), PPAR-gamma, calpain 10 (CAPN10) and genes coding for sex hormone binding globuline (SHBG), androgen receptor and insulin receptor substrate play an important role in the PCOS susceptibility (1). PCOS is a heterogenous disease and the genetic profile of different fenotypes may differ (5).

1.6 Environmental factors

Low birth weight is associated with an icreased risk of insulin resistance and diabetes mellitus type 2. Given the association between insulin resistance and hyperandrogenemia in patients with PCOS, low birth weight may therefore be associated with an increased risk for PCOS. Studies by Prof. Ibanez documented that girls that later developed PCOS had significantly lower birth weight than controls (7). However, in population studies low birth weight was associated with insulin resistance but not with hyperandrogenemia or with adrenal acitivity. These studies support that PCOS is not caused by low birth weight alone, but is more likely the result of interaction between genetic and environmental factors. There are speculations about influence of androgen exposure to development of fetal hyperandrogenic state (8). It is well known that lifestyle can modify PCOS phenotype. Environmental factors can be devided into the exogenous i.e. food, vitamin D deficiency, exposure to bisphenol A (PBA) - for example in study of Diamanti - Kadarakis PCOS women had significantly higher levels of PBA as compared to normal women (9). Among endogenous factors the most important are ethnicity, age, glycemia, insulin sennsitivity and many others.

1.7 Hyperinsulinemia and insulin resistance

The link between PCOS and insulin resistance was first described in 1980 and has later been confirmed in many studies. The exact mechanism of insulin resistance in patients with metabolic syndrome is however still unknown. Some patients have increased serine phosphorylation of beta subunit of insulin receptor but also distant parts of the insulin receptor cascade are affected (10). Some authors documented impaired glycogen synthase activity which was confirmed by studies on muscle biopsies from patients with PCOS. Impaired glucose metabolism in PCOS represents probably primary not secondary mechanism. Hyperinsulinaemia is frequently seen in obese PCOS but also in some lean PCOS women. Insulin sensitivity has been described to be reduced by 50% in lean PCOS patients which was statisticaly significant (11). Insulin stimulates p450c17 activity in ovaries and adrenals leading to increased androgen production. In addition, hyperinsulinemia decreases the hepatic SHBG production and through this mechanism free testosterone levels increases. Low SHBG is a good predictor of PCOS and is associated with impaired insulin sensitivity. The pathogenesis of PCOS may be looked as a vicious cycle involving both hyperandrogenaemia and insulin resistance/ hyperinsulinemia. Insulin resistance induces hyperinsulinemia and subsequently stimulates the ovarian and adrenal hormonal production, inhibits SHBG production and testosterone activity increases Figure3 (5).

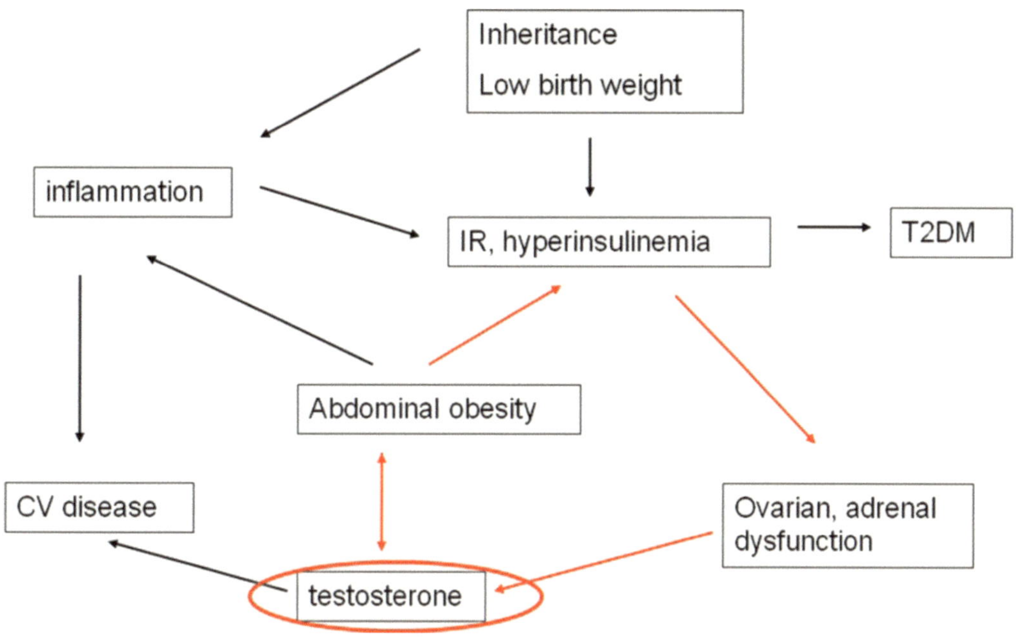

Fig. 3. Hyperinsulinemia and hyperandrogenemia as a vicious cycle in PCOS (5) CV-cardiovascular, IR insulin resistance, T2M – type 2 diabetes mellitus

Obesity and body fat distribution have an important influence on insulin sensitivity. Although 50% of PCOS women are not obese, obesity could potentially contribute to insulin resistance in PCOS. Lean PCOS women seem to have an insulin resistance that intrinsic to the syndrome, while in obese PCOS patients obesity additionally contributes to the impairment of the glucose metabolism (1). Elucidating the pathogenesis of insulin resistance in PCOS will provide insight into an important cause of type 2 diabetes (39).

Body composition and fat metabolism in PCOS

Approximately 75% patients with PCOS are overweight, but a high waist-to-hip ratio (WHR) indicating increased abdominal fat mass is seen in both normal and overweight patients with PCOS (5). There are only few studies concerning the correlations between phenotypic expression, body composition and PCOS, and relationship with the processes of growth and sexual maturation and various environmental factors (nutrition, physical activity, stress, and other factors). Variation in human body composition and shape ranges considerably: many body size and shape indices (height, weight, body composition, and proportions) are the result of long evolution process and adaptation to environment. Obviously, the morphological body parameters, physiological and biochemical indices are complex and compound the interdependent system. If waist circumference and WHR of women with PCOS increase, reproductive function and metabolic state of a woman is altered more than in cases when there are no changes in these parameters. The investigations of the strongest sexual dimorphism sign - the subcutaneous and visceral fat topography - showed that women with PCOS have greater adipose tissue mass in the areas of the abdomen, waist, and upper arms than control women (12).

Ghrelin and cholecystokinin secretion following meals are impaired in PCOS, suggesting changed appetite regulation. In a study of Glintborg et al. the prevalence of eating disorder was 36,3% in women presenting hirsutism, and controversely, PCOS was overrepresented in bulimic women (5). The genetic property of subclinical eating behaviour and the link between subclinical eating behaviour and PCOS has been studied before but the role of leptin within this connection has never been investigated. In the study of Jahanfar et al., serum leptin level correlated significantly with bulimia score. The genetic property of subclinical eating disorder was not confirmed. Leptin was linked with both subclinical eating disorder and PCOS (13).

In the study of Puder et al., PCOS women had significantly higher trunk to fat ratio (T/E fat) as compared with body mass index matched women, they also had higher values of inflammatory markers such as highly sensitive C-reactive protein (hsCRP), procalcitonin, tumor necrosis factor alpha (TNF-alpha). Additional adjusting to T/E fat eliminated the effect of PCOS on insulin resistance and inflammatory markers. They conclude that the increase in inflamatory markers in PCOS women is primarly associated with increased central fat excess rather than PCOS per se (14). Among other considerations, anomalies of plasma growth hormone (GH) secretion and/or altered insulin growth factor I (IGF-I) concentrations may play role in the pathogenesis of PCOS. Abdominal obesity, which can exacerbate the insulin resistance and reproductive features of the syndrome, is associated with profoundly reduced and disorderly GH secretion. A stimulatory role of GH in early and later stages of folliculogenesis and ovulation, hyposomatotropism may contribute to impaired follicular development and anovulation in PCOS (15). Increased intra-abdominal fat is of central importance in PCOS as it affects GH secretion, insulin resistance, lipid metabolism, and inflammatory status. Life style modification and weight loss improves ovulation rate and fertility and testosterone levels are decreased (5).

Inflammation

PCOS is a proinflamatory state as evidenced by elevated plasma concentrations of hsCRP. In obesity-related diabetic syndrome, TNF alpha is overexpressed in adipose tissue and induces insulin resistance through acute and chronic effects on insulin sensitive tissues. Chronic exposure to TNF-alfa decreases the expression of glucose transporter 4 (GLUT4), the insulin-sensitive glucose transport protein. Because decreased GLUT4 expression has been identified in PCOS, it is possible that TNFalpha contributes to this postreceptor defect.

The source of excess circulating TNFalpha in PCOS is likely to be adipose tissue in the obese. In lean women with PCOS increased visceral adiposity has been proposed as a source of excess TNFalpha (16).
Systemic review and metaanalysis of relevant studies suggest that adiponectin is lower in women with PCOS compared with non-PCOS controls of similar body mass index (BMI). Lower adiponectin levels are associated with the insulin resistance observed in women with PCOS compared with controls. It has been demonstrated that the more insulin resistant women with PCOS recruited, the lower serum adiponectin levels were found (17).
In PCOS previous studies showed positive associations between leptin and BMI, waist circumference and insulin resistance, indicating that fat mass in PCOS is the most important predictor of leptin secretion in PCOS and this data do not support a pathogenic role of leptin in PCOS. Chemokines such as migration inhibitor factor (MIF), monocyte chomatractant protein (MCP-1) and macrophage inflammatory protein (MIP) are increased and in some studies and well correlated with testosterone levels in PCOS patients (5, 16).

Cardiovascular risk factors in PCOS

High percentage of patients with PCOS have abnormal lipid profiles including increased total cholesterol (TC), low densitiy lipoprotein cholesterol (LDL-C), whereas high density cholesterol (HDL-C) levels are decreased. Patients with PCOS have increased prevalence of coronary atherosclerosis and echocardiography abnormalities but no prospective studies exist in PCOS populations. Retrospective studies found significantly increased risk of hypertension and cardiovascular disseases and current estimated risk for cardiovascular disseases is 4-11 fold increased in PCOS. Patients with PCOS have 5-7 fold higher risk for acute myocardial infarction, however no prospective studies exist until this time. There is increased CD36 which is expressed on the surface of monocytes and macrophages. In addition increased CD36, plasminogene activator inhibitor (PAI-1), homocystein were reported to be higher in women with PCOS. Previous studies did not found any differences in interleukin 6 (IL-6) between patients with PCOS and controls and no effect of metformin or glitazone treatment (1, 5). HsCRP is secreted in response to cytokines including IL-6. Despite the fact that data are inconsistent, increased levels of hsCRP in patients with PCOS were reported in some previous studies. HsCRP positively correlated with DEXA scan whereas no correlation was observed with testosterone levels. Pioglitazone-mediated improvement of insulin sensitivity was accompanied by decreased hsCRP levels (5, 18). Young women with PCOS mostly have a normal blood pressure, while especially older, obese patienst with PCOS suffer from an elevated blood pressure. In contrast to adolescent with PCOS who mostly have still normal lipid profiles, women with PCOS often have a dyslipidemia (1).

Risk of type 2 diabetes mellitus

PCOS is powerful risk factor for impaired glucose tolerance and type 2 diabetes mellitus. Insulin-resistant patients with PCOS maintain normal glucose levels by an insulin hypersecretion. These patients are at an icreased risk of beta cell exhaustion and development of type 2 diabetes mellitus (19). In study of women with PCOS the prevalance of diabetes mellitus was up to 7,5% and impaired glucose tolerance was 31% (1,20). Metaanalysis of clinical studies has been performed by Moran et al. Totaly 2 192 studies were reviewed and 35 were selected for final analysis. Results showed an increased prevalence of impaired glucose tolerance and type 2 diabetes mellitus and metabolic syndrome in both BMI and non BMI-matched studies Table 2 (21).

	OR non BMI	BMI-matched
IGT	2,48	2,58
DMt2	4,43	4,0
MS	2,88	2,2

Table 2. Prevalence of impaired glucose tolerance (IGT) and type 2 diabetes mellitus (DMt2) and metabolic syndrome (MS) in BMI and non BMI-matched studies (21)

Other risks of PCOS

Among risks related to pregnancy there was documented a higher prevalence of gestational diabetes mellitus, which was significantly higher than that in control group of women. Moreover, patients with PCOS have significantly higher risk of pregnancy-induced hypertension, preeclampsia, neonatal complications and higher abortrtion rate. Women with PCOS seem to expierence increased risk of cesarean delivery and perinatal morbidity and mortality (22). There is also increased risk of breast cancer as well as endometrial cancer (33).

Bone mineral density (BMD) in PCOS

Several factors may contribute to the conserved BMD in PCOS. Patients with PCOS have relatively high levels of estradiol and are characterized by abdominal obesity and insulin resistance. Abdominal obesity and increased visceral fat mass are seen in overweight and normal-weight patients with PCOS. Adiposity is known to be positively associated with BMD. Furthermore, more than 50% of patients with PCOS are insulin resistant, and previous studies suggested that hyperinsulinemia, independent of BMI, may protect against the development of osteoporosis. Only few studies found positive associations between testosterone and BMD in PCOS, but this may in part be explained by the use of imprecise testosterone assays in most studies (23). In the study of Glintborg, treatment with pioglitazone of insulin-resistant premenopausal patients with PCOS was followed by significantly decreased BMD at the hip and lumbar spine and decreased markers of bone mineral turnover. These findings suggest that pioglitazone may have adverse effects on BMD even in a study population relatively protected from bone mineral loss (23).

Vitamin D and PCOS

Recent studies clearly documented that obesity is associated with decreased 25OH vitamin D levels. Patients with PCOS and metabolic syndrome had significantly lower levels of vitamin D2 being in negative correlation with fasting insulin and insulin sensitivity. Supporting the relative vitamin D insuficiency in PCOS some studies found a higher levels of parathormone (PTH) in these patients. Association between vitamin D receptor (VDR) gene polymorphisms (Apal) and insulin resistance, PTH, 25OH vitamin D is speculated. Some authors documented efficacy of vitamin D replacement on insulin resistance and in the treatmend of anovulation (24, 25, 26). Low serum 25OH vitamin D concentrations result from the presence of obesity and insulin resistance (24).

In the study of Wehr et al., the prevalance of vit D deficiency in 206 women affected by PCOS was 72.8%. PCOS women with metabolic syndrome had lower vit D levels than PCOS women without metabolic symptoms. In multivariate regression analysis 25OHD and BMI were independent predictors of homeostatic model assessment-insulin resistance index (HOMA), vitamin D was also independent predictor of metabolic syndrome in PCOS. There was significant positive correlation of vitamin D levels SHBG and quantitative insulin sensitivity check index (QUICKI) and a negative one found with BMI, WHR, waist circumference, blood pressure, glucose, isnulin, HOMA-IR and triglycerides. Nevertheless large intervetion trial are needed to evaluate the effect of vit D supplementation on metabolic distubances in PCOS Table 3 (27).

Positive correlation of 25OHD

SHBG	0,009

Negative correlations of 25OHD

Waist circumference	0,001
Hip circumference	0,001
Blood pressure	0,05
Fasting glucose	0,001
Fasting insulin	0,001
HOMA IR	0,001
Triglycerides	0,002
CRP	0,005

Table 3. Correlations of vitamin 25OHD (27)

Autoimmunity and PCOS

There are some reports regarding the relationship between PCOS and autoimmune disorders. However, the data are controversial and some studies documented a higher prevalence of antihistone and anti ds-DNA antibodies in PCOS (28). Concerning organ-specific antibodies, one study clearly demonstrated a high prevalence of antibodies against thyroid specific components, higher prevalence of autoimmune thyroiditis and higher thyrotropin levels as well (29). There are so far no reports about antiovarian antibodies in patients with PCOS. There are speculations about the presence of antivorian simulating antibodies analogically to thyroid simulating antibodies (28). As was documented by the study of Janssen and colleagues, patients with PCOS had significantly higher frequency of antihyroid antibodies and ultrasound picture hypoechogenic thyroid gland (29).

2. Diagnosis of PCOS

Diagnostic approach in PCOS includes:

1. History taking and physical examination
2. Laboratory and hormonal evaluations
3. Ovarian ultrasonography

Physical examination includes: assessment of hirsutism using scoring scale of Feriman and Gallwey, measurment of blood pressure, waist and hip ratio.

Transvaginal ultrasonography is necessary to confirm polycystic ovaries.
Laboratory investigations include: total and free testosterone, SHGB, LH, FSH, prolactin, 17hydroxy-progesterone, dehydroepiandrosterone sulfate (DHEAS), fasting plasma glucose and lipids, TSH.
Secondary evaluation includes exclusion of suspected Cushing syndrome: 24 hours UFC, Dexamethasone supression test (overnight, 2 mg 2 days), oral glucose tolerance test if fasting blood glucose is between 5,6 - 7,0 mmol/l and magnetic resonance (computer tomography) of adrenal glands – if suspected virillizing tumor.

3. Treatment of PCOS

Various intervetions have been proposed ranging from life-style modifications, administration of pharmaceutical agents (such as clomiphene citrate, insulin sensitizing agents, gonadotropins and gonadotropin-releasing hormone analogues), the use of laparoscopic ovarian drilling and the application of assisted reproduction techniques (30).
Treatment is related to the preference of patient and includes:

1. Treatment of hirsutism or acne
2. Treatment of oligo/amenorrhea and infertility
3. Treatment of insulin resistance and metabolic syndrome

1. Treatment of hirsutism or acne

Combination of estrogene-progestin therapy in the form of ***oral contraceptives*** is the first line of endocrine treatment for hirsutism and acne. The estrogenic component is responsible for the supression of LH and thus serum androgen levels. It also results in increase of SHBG lowering the free fraction of testosterone. Assessment of adequacy of ovarian suppression can be made at the end of the third week after starting treatment. The effect on acne can be expected to be maximal in 1-2 months. However, the effect on hair growth may not be evident for 6 months and the maximum effect requires 9-12 months (31). ***Cyproterone acetate*** acts by competitive inhibition of the binding of testosterone and dihydrotestosterone to the androgen receptors. ***Spironolactone*** appears to be as effective an antiandrogen as cyproterone actetate in doses 100-200 mg daily. ***Flutamide*** is a potent nonsteroidal antiandrogen without progestational, estrogenic, corticoid, antigonadotropic effect (32, 33). ***Finasteride*** is a competitive inhibitor of type 2 5alpha-reductase and for this reason can be useful for the treatment of hirsutism (33, 34).
Gonadotropin-releasing hormone agonists *(GnRH agonists)* have been reported to be effective in the treatment of hirsutism. Their chronic administration supresses pituitary-ovarian function thus inhibiting both ovarian androgen and estrogen secretion. Addition of dexamethasone to leuprolide has been reported to further improve the response in some women with PCOS (33).
Recent randomized, prospecitve trial comparing low dose flutamide, finasteride, ketoconazole and combination cyproterone-acetate-ethinyl estradiol demonstrated relative superiority of flutamide and cyproterone acetate-ethinyl estradiol in the treatment of hirsutism (33).
Aims of treatment hirsutism or acne include:

- suppression of adrenal or ovarian androgen production
- alteration of binding of androgens to their plasma proteins
- impairment of the peripheral conversion of androgen precursors to active androgen
- inhibition of androgen action in peripheral tissues

2. Treatment of oligo/amenorrhea and infertility

Chronic oligoanovulation results in persistent stimulation of endometrial tissue by estrogen increasing the risk of endometrial cancer. A three-fold increased risk of endometrial cancer has been reported. Thus anovulatory women with PCOS are recommended to take progestins to reduce the risk of endometrial hyperplasia or carcinoma. The combined estrogene-progestin therapy is also beneficial in women with PCOS because in both inhibits endometrial proliferation and reduces ovarian androgen production (33). In some studies insulin sensitizing agents such as metformin and glitazone improved menstrual cycle irregularities, however their indication in case when patient does not wish to be pregnant is controversial and generally not recommended (30).

Clomiphene citrate remains still the first line therapy for induction of ovulation in women with PCOS. The usual regimen is 50 mg per day for 5 days beginning on cycle day 3 mg daily for 5 days, ovulation can be induced in about 80% of women (33). There are many reports about combined clomiphene citrate and metformin therapy, unfortunately with controversial results. In higher doses metformin together with clomiphene citrate significantly improved ovulation rate and pregnancy rate, however did not improved live birth rate. Those patients who fail clomiphene therapy will usually require either low dose human recombinant FSH or human menoapusal gonadotropin for ovulation induction. Pregnancy rate is similar to clomiphene citrate, but live birth rate is lower when compared with clomiphene citrate (30, 35, 36).

There has been renewed interest in surgically inducing ovulation in women with PCOS using laparoscopy and electrocautery or laser. Laparoscopic ovarian diathermy (LOD) is associated with lower multiple gestation rates than gonadotropins, because LOD can achieve unifollicular ovulation. There was no evidence of difference in live birth rate and miscarriage in women with clomiphene-resistant PCOS undergoing LOD versus gonadotropin treatment. LOD is an alternative to gonadotropin therapy for clomiphene-citrate resistant anovulatory PCOS. LOD restores menstrual regularity in 63%-85% of women, and the benefitial effects on reproductive outcomes seem to last for several years in many women (30, 37).

Progestins: reduce risk of endometrial cancer

Estrogene-progestin: inhibits endometrial proliferation, reduces androgen production

Clomiphene citrate: first line therapy (80% ovulation rate)

Human recombinant FSH: if clomiphene failed

Human menopausal gonadotropin

Aromatase inhibitors

Surgically induced ovulation: laparoscopy, electrocautery, laser (80% pregnancy rate, 80% conceptions within first 8 months)

In vitro fertilization

3. Treatment of insulin resistance and metabolic syndrome

Insulin resistance in women with PCOS appears more common than in the general population. Many studies show the common coexistence of obesity with insulin resistance, particulary in the presence of abdominal phenotype, although this disorder may be present even in those with normal weight. PCOS-related insulin resistance is partly independent of the presence of obesity, and that obesity in PCOS women simply adds and additional deterious effects on insulin sensitivity, by mechanisms that have still not been defined and could be different between obese and non-obese PCOS women (38). In women with PCOS, basal insulin secretion is increased and hepatic insulin clearance is reduced, resulting in hyperinsulinemia. Obesity and PCOS have a synergistic negative impact on insulin senzitivity. In both obese and non-obese PCOS women , insulin secretion is inappropriately low for their degree od insulin resistance, suggesting the presence of pancreatic beta-cell dysfunction. There is a positive association between insulin and androgen levels in their PCOS subjects (39). Insulin resistance also appears to play a pathogenic role in the metabolic syndrome. Metabolic syndrome and its components are common in women with PCOS, placing them at increased risk for cardiovascular disease (40). Women with PCOS have 11-fold increase in the prevalence of metabolic syndrome compared with age-matched controls (41).

As noted, lowering insulin levels with weight reduction or drugs may induce ovulation in obese, hyperinsulinemic women with PCOS. Weight loss prior to improves live birth rate in obese women with or without PCOS. Multiple observation studies have noted that weight loss is associated with improved spontaneous ovulation rates in women with PCOS, while pregnancies have been reported after losing as little as 5% of initial body weight. However weight loss is recommended for those who are overweight with a body mass index over 25-27 kg/m2 (30, 33).

Insulin resistance is regarded as a major pathophysiological feature of the syndrome. Therefore, agents that improve insulin sensitivity, that is, metformin ant thiazolidinediones (TZDs), have been extensively trialled in PCOS patients with encouraging results (42).

Metformin treatment and PCOS

Metformin is a biguanide agent used in the treatment of type 2 diabetes mellitus. In women with PCOS, metformin was sparked by the recognition of its pleiotropic actions on several tissues. It lowers serum insulin levels and improves insulin sensitivity not only by its glucose lowering effect but also by increasing peripheral glucose utilization. Apart from its action on classic insulin-sensitive tissues, it has been clearly demonstrated that metformin has a positive effect in the treatment of reproductive abberations in women with PCOS, which indirectly suggests a potential direct effect at the ovarian level. Metformin treatment increases ovulation rate, improves menstrual cyclicity, and reduces serum androgen levels in these patients (38). Metformin appears to affect ovarian function in a dual mode through the elevation of insulin excess acting upon the ovary and through direct ovarian effects. Regarding the action of metformin on theca cells, data demonstrate reduced CYP17 activity in women with PCOS. In rat granulosa cells, metformin treatment was shown to reduce basal and FSH-stimulated progesterone and estradiol production (43). Metformin may exert a direct effect on granulosa cells through activation of 5´-adenosine monophosphate activated protein kinase (AMPK) and subsequent reduction of steroid production (44). Stimulation of AMPK appears to be a key mediator of metformin´s action on hepatic gluconeogenesis and lipogenesis (43). The analysis of follicular fluid seemed to confirm that metformin acts directly on the ovary improving local levels of androgens, ovarian insulin resistance and the levels of several growth factors, Figure 4 (52).

Metformin restores ovulation in a significant proportion of patients with PCOS and has resulted in pregnancy. Metformin pretreatment improves the efficacy of clomiphene-citrate on PCOS patients with clomiphene-citrate resistance (19, 33). The target dose is 1500-2550 mg/day. Clinical response is usually seen at the dose of 1000 mg daily (33). Recent small studies also suggest that metformin continued during pregnancy reduces the high rates of gestational diabetes and first-trimester spontaneous abortion characteristic of PCOS (19, 43). Some studies have reported a decrease in TC, LDL-C and triglyceride levels and increase in

HDL-C concentration whereas others have not. Another study in its metaanalysis found only LDL-C levels to be significantly reduced following metformin treatment, with TC, HDL-C a triglyceride remaining unchanged (44). Metformin has been shown to exert antiatheroslerotic, anti-inflmatory and antithrombotic properties by reducing carotic intima-media thickness, endothelin, hsCRP, PAI-1 and leptin and increasing adiponectin levels in PCOS patients (42). Metformin treatment has been associated with decreased androgen (total and free testosterone, androstendione) and LH levels and increased SHBG and DHEAS concentrations (42).

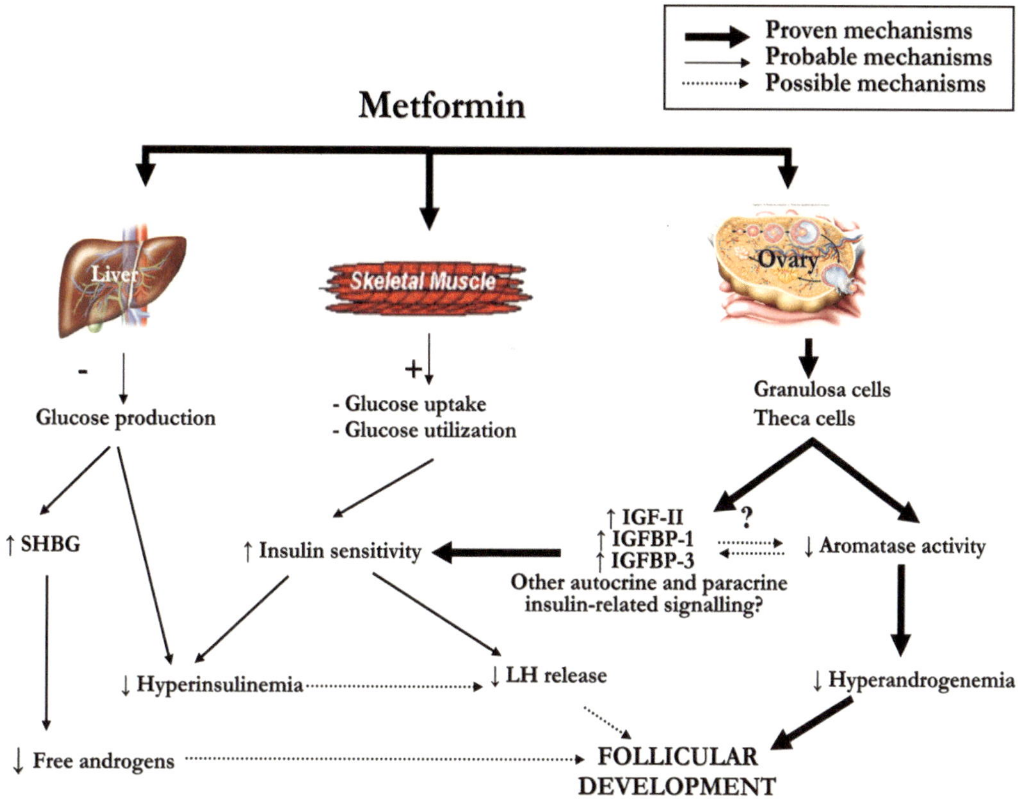

Fig. 4. Hypothesis for metformin effects on follicular development (52)

Knowledge regarding the predictors for metformin response is crucial. Some studies demonstrated that metformin appears to benefit to PCOS subjects irrespective of their weight or degree of insulin resistance. Metformin may be more effective in insulin-resistance PCOS patients with low BMI. There have been examinated genetic factors. Polymorphism of serine-threonine kinase gene STK11 was associated with a significantly decreased chance of ovulation in PCOS subjects treated with metformin (38). It is commonly expierence that obese women, particulary those with morbid obesity, are refractory to metformin therapy. Insulin resistant PCOS patients with low BMI were reported to be more likely to respond to metformin. However, previous studies did not confirm the predictive value of insulin resistance indices for ovulation induction by metformin. Metformin may be able to directly affect ovarian steroidogenesis. This drug could affect the central regulation of ovulation by modulating GnRH release through the activation of the hypothalamic AMPK (43). The study of Palomba et al. demonstrates that the efficacy of metformin in inducing ovulation in patients with polycystic ovary syndrome is probably due to a direct action of the drug on the ovary, and that the ovulatory response to the drug seems to be related more to local drug sensitivity or resistance than to improvements in the systemic hormonal and/or metabolic pattern (52). Treating insulin resistance with metformin may improve fertility, facilitate weight loss, improve the lipid profile, reduce the incidence of diabetes, and prevent atherosclerosis, myocardial infarction, and stroke (19). It is very difficult to conclude regarding the efficacy of metformin in PCOS, since the published data are incosistent due to various study designs concerning patients characteristics, weight change, dose regimen and outcome meassures.

TZDs are ligands of the peroxisome proliferator-activator receptor-gamma, a nuclear transcription factor. TZDs lower fasting and postprandial glucose levels by increasing glucose utilization in skeletal muscle and decreasing hepatic gluconeogenesis and ameliorate hypertiglyceridemia (38, 42). In PCOS patients, rosiglitazone treatment improved insulin resistance and normalized the menstrual cycle (45). It had beneficial effect on serum levels of adipinectin and resistin (46). Rosiglitazone decreased fastig glucose and insulin levels, increase HDL-C and reduced TC and LDL-C and triglyceride concentration (42). Tarkun et al. observed that rosiglitazone treatment decreased androgen production and it had benefecial effects on endothelian dysfunction and low-grade chronic inflammation in normal weight women with PCOS (47). In another study, rosiglitazone therapy decreased androgen levels (DHEAS, total and free testosterone), increase SHBG levels, reduced estradiol production and restored menstrual cycles, induced ovulation rate and improved hirsutism score (42). Rosiglitazone has been shown to enhance both sponateneous and clomiphene-induced ovulation in overweight and obese women with PCOS (37,48). However, due to its side effect, it has been withdrawn from the market. The efficacy of rosiglitazone and pioglitazone in PCOS has not been compared in any study (42).

Administration of pioglitazone in women with PCOS resulted in remarkable decline in fasting serum insulin levels, improvement of insulin sensitivity. Pioglitazone increased serum SHBG concentrations, resulting in significant decrease in the free androgen index. Treatment was also associated with higher ovulation rates (49). In women with PCOS who failed to respond optimally to meformin, when pioglitazone was added, insulin, glucose, insulin resistance, insulin secretion, and DHEAS fell, HDL-C, TC and SHBG rose, and menstrual regularity improved (50). Application of insulin sensitizers showed favorable influence on the basic hormonal deviations in PCOS - the hyperandrogenemia and insulin resistance. In cases with PCOS, metformin treatment influences better hyperandrogenemia, while rosiglitazone affects more pronouncedly insulin resistance and hyperinsulinemia (51). The study of Li et al. included meta-analysis of 10 trials. TZDs were found to be superior to metformin in reducing serum levels of free testosterone and DHEAS after 3-month treatment. Decreases in triglyceride levels were more pronounced with metformin after 6 months. Decreases in BMI are greater with metformin treatment as assessed at 3 and 6 months. The findings do not indicate that metformin is superior to TZDs for the treatment of PCOS or vice versa. Between studies, heterogeneity was a major confounder (53).

TZDs should be used in substitution of or in adition to metformin in insulin-resistant or obese PCOS women who do not tolerate or do not respond to metformin therapy. For menstrual disorders, oral contraceptives are considered the primary treatment, with intermittent progesterone therapy and insulin-sensitizing agents as alternative therapies (38, 42).

4. Conclusions

PCOS is a common disorder which affects 5%-10% of women of reproductive age (1). PCOS can be described as a multiorgan disease affecting most endocrine organs including ovaries, adrenals, pituitary, fat cells, bones, and endocrine pancreas (5). However, the diagnosis of PCOS comprises more than reproductive or cosmetics problems Table 4. PCOS constitutes major health issue for young women. Insulin resistance, dyslipidemia and hypertension contribute to an enhanced cardiovascular and diabetes risk (1).

Adolescents	Reproductive phase	Postmenopause
Oligomenorrhea	Infertility	Impaired glucose tolerance
Hirsutism	Hirsutism	Type 2 diabetes
Acne	Obesity	Dyslipidemia
Obesity	Impaired glucose tolerance	Hypertension
		Cardiovaskular risk factors

Table 4. PCOS throughout the life cycle (1)

The risk of diabetes is greater in anovulatory women with polycystic ovaries, in obese subjects and those with a family history of type 2 diabetes (3). Women with PCOS are at significantly increased risk for impaired glucose tolerance and type 2 diabetes (31,1% impaired glucose tolerance, 7,5% undiagnosed diabetes) (20, 21). Legro et al. found that not only obese but also nonobese PCOS women may also have glucose intolerance (10,3% impaired glucose tolerance, 1,5% diabetes) (20). Abdominal obesity appears to be the primary determinant of metabolic abnormalities in PCOS (2). Abdominal obesity and increased activation of the inflammatory system are seen in both normal weight and obese patients with PCOS. (5). Subclinical inflammation and insulin resistance are important predictors of cardiovaslular disease. Patients with PCOS have an excess of central fat independent of total fat mass. Central fat excess is usually associated with an increase in serum inflammatory markers and insulin resistance. On the other hand, sex hormones affect body fat distribution and thereby might in part explain the genderspecific differences in body fat distribution (14). Insulin resistance and hyperandrogenism may also, either directly or indirectly, influence metabolic abnormalities and potentially contribute to abdominal obesity (2). Abdominal obesity and insulin resistance stimulate ovarian and adrenal androgen production, whereas SHBG levels are decreased (5). Women with PCOS should be informed of their long-term risk of type 2 diabetes and likely cardiovascualr disease. There is need for a comperhensive screening and education program for women of all ages with PCOS (41). While hyperandrogenemia and concomitant hirsutism, acne, or infertility are certainly troublesome to a woman, an incereased risk of developing diabetes and atherosclerosis has the potential to shorten her lifespan (19).

PCOS is a unique, natural model for the study of influence of androgen excess on bone mass among women. The deleterious effect on bone of amenorrhea is balanced by androgen overproduction. Obesity and insulin resistance aggravate hyperandrogenism. Serum vitamin D is significantly lower in obese than in non-obese women individuals and may contribute to lower serum 25OH vitamin D in obesity. Hypovitaminosis D results from the presence of obesity but is independent of the presence of PCOS. Vitamin D supplementation can be useful in the treatment of obese women with PCOS (24). Wehr et al. are the first to describe an inverse association of low 25OH vitamin D levels with impaired beta-cell function, impaired glucose tolerance, and metabolic syndrome in women with PCOS (27).

The treatment of infertile women with PCOS is surrounded by many controversies. Before any intervention is initiated, the improvement of life-style, especially weigh reduction is recomended. Clomiphene-citrate, an anti-estrogen remains the first-line of treatment for ovulation induction. Recomended second-line of intervetion is eihter exogenous gonadotropins or laparoscopic ovarian surgery. Recomended third-line treatment is *in vitro* fertilization (30). Treating of insulin resistance, when present, with metformin may improve fertility, facilitate weight loss, improve the lipid profile, reduce the incidence of diabetes, and prevent atherosclerosis, myoacrdial infarction, and stroke (19). The use of metformin alone or in combination with life-style modifications has produced a list of metabolic and clinical benefits in both obese and non-obese women with PCOS which has allowed an indiscriminate use of this compound worldwide (38). On the other hand, according to ESHRE/ASRM-Sponsored PCOS Consensus Workshop Group metformin use in PCOS should be restricted to women with glucose intolerance (30). According to Nestler metformin remains an important therapeutic option in the pharmacologic treatment of infertility in PCOS, and its use should not be restricted to women with glucose intolerance, as recomended by the ESHRE/ASRM Consensus statement (35).

Because of the high prevalence of PCOS and the long-term implications on metabolic risk factors, fertility, and quality of life, doctors need to be aware of the syndrome in daily practise (5). In conclusion, it is clear that PCOS is an anigma. Its underlying pathophysiology is not fully understood. No treatment is a panacea, because treatments, so far, have been directed at the symptoms but not at the syndrome itself (33).

5. References

[1] Schroder AK, Tauchert S, Ortmann O, Diedrich K, Weiss JM. Insulin resistance in patients with polycystic ovary syndrome. Ann Med 2004; 36: 426-439

[2] Moran L, Teede H. Metabolic features of the reproductive phenotypes of polycystic ovary syndrome. Hum Reprod 2009; 15: 477-488

[3] The Rotterdam ESHRE/ASRM - sponsored PCOS consensus workshop group. Revised 2003 consensus on diagnostic criteria and longterm health risks related to polycystic ovary syndrome (PCOS). Hum Reprod 2004; 19, 41-47

[4] Burt Solorzano CM, McCarteney CR, Blank SK, Knudsen KL, Marshall JC. Hyperandrogenemia in adolescent girls: origins of abnormal gonadotropin-releasing hormone secretion. BJOG 2010; 117: 143-149

[5] Glintborg D, Andersen M. An update on the pathogenesis, inflammation, and metabolism in hirsutism and polycystic ovary syndrome. Gynecol Endocrinol 2010; 26: 281-296

[6] Franks S, Webber LJ, Goh M, Valentine A, White DM, Conway GS, Wiltshire S, McCarthy MI. Ovarian morphology is a marker of heritable biochemical traits in sisters with polycystic ovaries. J Clin Endocrinol Metab 2008; 93, 3396-3402

[7] Ibánez L, Vall C, Potau N, Marcos MV, de Zegher F. Polycystic ovary syndrome after precocious pubarche: ontogeny of low-birthweight effect. Clin Endocrinol 2001; 55: 667-672
[8] Nisenbalt V, Norman RJ. Androgens and polycystic ovary syndrome. Curr Opin Endocrinol Diabetes Obes 2009; 16: 224-231
[9] Kandaraki E, Chatzigeorgiou A, Livadas S, Palioura E, Economou F, Koutsilieris M, Palimeri S, Panidis D, Diamanti-Kadarakis E. Endocrine disruptors and polycystic ovary syndrome (PCOS): elevated serum levels of bisphenol A in women with PCOS. J Clin Endocrinol Metab 2011; 96: 480-484
[10] Auchus RJ, Geller DH, Lee TC, Miller Wl. The regulation of human P450c17 activity: relationship to premature adrenarche, insulin resistance and polycystic ovary syndrome. Trends Endocrinol Metab 1998; 9: 47-50
[11] Morales AJ, Laughlin GA, Butzow T, Maheswari H, Baumann G, Zen SS. Insulin, somatotropic, and luteinizing hormone axes in lean and obese women with polycystic ovary syndrome: common and distinct features. J Clin Endocrinol Metab 1996; 8: 2854-2864
[12] Zabuliene L, Tutkuviene J. Body compossition and polycystic ovary syndrome. Medicina (Kaunas) 2010; 46: 142-157
[13] Jahanfar Sh, Maleki H, Mosavi AR. Subclinical eating disorder, polycystic ovary syndrome - is there any connection between these two conditions throuhg leptin - a twin study. Med J Malaysia 2005; 60: 441-446
[14] Puder JJ, Varga S, Kraenzlin M, De Geyter Ch, Keller U, Muller B. Central fat excess in polycystic ovary syndrome: relation to low-grade inflammation and insulin resistance. J Clin Endocrinol Metab 2005; 90:6014-6021
[15] Van Dam EWCM, Roelfsema F, Helmerhorst FM, Frolich M, Meinders AE, Veldhuis JD, Pilj H. Low amplitude and disordely spontaneous growth hormone releasing in obese women with or without polycystic ovary syndrome. J Clin Endocrinol Metab 2002; 87: 4225-4230
[16] Gonzáles F, Minium J, Rote NS, Kirwan JP. Hyperglycemia alters tumor necrosis factor-alpfa release from mononuclear cells in women with polycystic ovary syndrome. J Clin Endocrinol Metab 2005; 90: 5336-5342
[17] Toulis KA, Goulis DG, Farmakiotis D, Georgopoulos NA, Katsikis I, Tarlatzis BC, Papadimas I, Panidis D. Adiponectin levels in women with polycystic ovary syndrome: a systematic review and meta-analysis. Hum Reprod 2009; 15: 297-307
[18] Tosi F, Dorizzi R, Castello R, Maffeis C, Spiazzi G, Zoppini G, Muggeo M, Moghetti P. Body fat insulin resistance independently predict increased serum C-reactive protein in hyperandrogenic women with polycystic ovary syndrome. Eur J Endocrinol 2009; 161: 737-45
[19] Goodarzi MO, Korenman SG. The importance of insulin resistance in polycystic ovary syndrome. Fertil Steril 2003; 80: 255-258
[20] Legro RS, Kunselman AR, Dodson WC, Dunaif A. Prevalence and predictors of risk for type 2 diabetes mellitus and impaired glucose toelrance in polycystic ovary syndrome: a prospective, controlled study in 254 affected women. J Clin Endocrinol Metab 1999; 84: 165-169

[21] Moran L, Misso ML, Wild RA, Norman RJ. Impaired glucose tolerance, type 2 diabetes and metabolic syndrome in polycystic ovary syndrome: a review and meta-analysis. Hum Reprod 2010; 4: 347-363
[22] Lavazzo C, Vitoratos N. Polycystic ovarian syndrome and pregnancy outcome. Arch Gynecol Obstet 2010; 282:235-239
[23] Glintborg D, Andersen M, Hagen C, Heickendorff L, Hermann AP. Association of pioglitazone treatment with decreased bone mineral density in obese premenopausal patients with polycystic ovary syndrome: a randomized, placebo-controlled trial. J Clin Endocrinol Metab 2008; 93: 1696-1701
[24] Yildizhan R, Kurdoglu M, Adali E, Kolusari A, Yildizhan B, Sahim HG, Kamaci M. Serum 25-hydroxyvitamin D concentrations in obese and non-obese women with polycystic ovary syndrome. Arch Gynecol Obstet 2009; 280: 559-563
[25] Selimoglu H, Durac C, Kiyici S, Ersoy C, Guclu M, Ozkaya G, Tuncel E, Erturk E, Imamoglu S. The effect of vitamin D replacement therapy on insulin resistance and androgen levels in women with polycystic ovary syndrome. J Endocrinol Invest 2010; 33: 234-238
[26] Mahmoudi T. Genetic variation in the vitamin D receptor and polycystic ovary syndrome. Fertil Steril 2009; 92: 1381-1383
[27] Wehr E, Pliz S, Schweighofer N, Giuliani A, Kopera D, Pieber TR, Obermayer-Pietsch B. Association of hypovitaminosis D with metabolic disturbances in polycystic ovary syndrome. E J Endocrinol 2009; 161 575-582
[28] Petríková J, Lazúrová I, Shoenfeld Y. Polycystic ovary syndrome and autoimmunity. E J Int Med 2010; 21: 369-371
[29] Janssen OE, Mehlmauer N, Hahn S, Offner AH, Gartner R. High prevalence of autoimmune thyroiditis in patients with polycystic ovary syndrome. Eur J Endocrinol 2004; 150: 363-369
[30] The Thessaloniki ESHRE/ASRM-sponsored PCOS Consensus workshop group. Consensus of infertility treatment related to polycystic ovary syndrome. Hum Reprod 2008; 23: 462-477
[31] Saha L, Kaur S, Saha PK. Pharmacotherapy of polycystic ovary syndrome - an update. Fundam Clin Pharmacol 2011; 7
[32] Karakurt F, Sahin I, Guler S, Demirbas B, Culha C, Serter R, Aral Y, Bavbek N. Comparison of the clinical efficacy of flutamide and spironolactone plus ethinyloestradiol/cyproterone acetate in treatment of hirsutism: a randomized controlled study. Adv Ther 2008; 25: 321-328
[33] Badway A, Elnshar A. Treatment options for polycystic ovary syndrome. I J Women´s Health; 2011 3: 25-35
[34] Lakryc EM, Motta EL, Soares JM, Haidar MA, Lima GR, Baracat EC. The benefits of finasteride for hirsutism women with polycystic ovary syndrome or idiopathic hirsutism. Gynecol Endocrinol 2003; 17: 57-63
[35] Nestler JE. Metformin in the treatment of infertility in PCOS: an alternative perspective. Fertil Steril 2008; 90: 14-16
[36] Legro RS, Barnhart HX, Schlaff WD, Carr BR, Diamond MP, Carson SA, Steinkampf MP, Coutifaris C, McGovern PG, Cataldo NA, Gosman GG, Nestler JE, Giudice LC.

Clomiphene, metformin, or both for infertility in the polycystic ovary syndrome. N Engl J Med 2007 356: 551-566
[37] Al-Fadhli R, Tulandi T. Laparoscopic treatment of polycystic ovaries: is its place diminidhing? Curr Opin Obstet Gynecol 2004; 16: 295-298
[38] Pasquali R, Gambineri A. Targeting insulin sensitivity in the treatment of polycystic ovary syndrome. Expert Opin Ther Targets 2009; 13: 1205-1226
[39] Venkatesan AM, Dunaif A, Corbould A. Insulin resistance in polycystic ovary syndrome: progress and paradoxes. Recent prog res 2001; 56: 295-308
[40] Apridonidze T, Essah PA, Iuorno MJ, Nestler JE. Prevalence and characteristics of the metabolic syndrome in women with polycystic ovary syndrome. J Clin Endocrinol Metabl 2005; 90: 1929-1935
[41] Dokras A, Bochner M, Hollinrake E, Markham S, VanVoorhis B, Jagasia DH. Screening women with polycystic ovary syndrome for metabolic syndrome. Obstet Gynecol 2005; 106: 131-137
[42] Katsiki N, Hatzitolios A. Insulin-sensitizing agents in the treatment of polycystic ovary syndrome: an update. Curr Opin Obstet Gynecol 2010; 22: 466-476
[43] Diamanti-Kandarakis E, Christakou ChD, Kandaraki E, Economou N. Metformin: an old medication of new fashion: evolving new molecular mechanisms and clinical implications in polycystic ovary syndrome. E J Endocrinol 2010; 162: 193-212
[44] Diamanti-Kandarakis E, Economou F, Palimeri S, Christakou Ch. Metformin in polycystic ovary syndrome. Ann NY Sci 2010; 1205: 192-198
[45] Belli SH, Graffigna MN, Oneto A, Otero P, Schurman L, Levalle OA. Effect of rosiglitazone on insulin resistance, growth factors, and reproductive disturbances in women with polycystic ovary syndrome. Fertil Steril 2004; 81: 624-629
[46] Majuri A, Santaniemi M, Rautio K, Kunnari A, Vartainen J, Ruokonen A, Kesaniemi YA, Tapanainen JS, Ukkola O, Morin-Papunen L. Rosiglitazone treatment increases plasma levels of adiponectin and decreases levels of resistin in overweight women with PCOS: a randomized placebo-controlled study. E J Endocrinol 2007; 156: 263-269
[47] Tarkun I, Cetinarslan B, Turemen E, Sahin T, Canturk Z, Komsuoglu B. Effect of rosiglitazone in insulin resistance, C-reactive protein and endothelial function in non-obese young women with polycystic ovary syndrome. E J Endocrinol 2005; 153: 115-121
[48] Ghazeeri G, Kutteh WH, Bryer-Ash M, Haas D, Ke RW. Effect of rosiglitazone on spontaneous and clomiphene citrate-induced ovulation in women with polycystic ovary syndrome. Fertil Steril 2003; 79: 562-566
[49] Brettenthaler N, DeGeyter Ch, Humer PR, Keller U. Effect of the insulin sensitizer pioglitazone on insulin resistance, hyperandrogenism, and ovulatory dysfunction in women with polycystic ovary syndrome. J Clin Endocrinol Metab 2004; 89: 3835-3840
[50] Glueck ChJ, Moreira A, Goldenberg N, Sieve L, Wang P. Pioglitazone and metformin in obese women with polycystic ovary syndrome not optimally responsive to metformin. Hum Reprod 2003; 18: 1618-1625
[51] Mitkov M, Pehlivanov B, Terzieva D. Metformin versus rosiglitazone in the treatment of polycystic ovary syndrome. E J Obstet Gynecol 2006; 126: 93-98

[52] Palomba S, Falbo A, Russ T, Orio F, Tolino A, Zullo F. Systemic and local effects of metformin administration in patients with polycystic ovary syndrome (PCOS): relationship to the ovulatory response. Hum Reprod 2010; 25: 1005-1013

[53] Li XJ, Zu YX, Liu CQ, Zhang W, Zhang HJ, Zan B, Wang LY, Zang SY, Zhang SH. Metformin vs thiazolidinediones for treatment of clinical, hormonal and metabolic characteristics of polycystic ovary syndrome: a meta-analysis. Cliin Endocrinol (Oxf) 2011; 74:332- -339

5

Management Approaches to Congenital Adrenal Hyperplasia in Adolescents and Adults; Latest Therapeutic Developments

Gül Bahtiyar and Alan Sacerdote
Woodhull Medical and Mental Health Center, SUNY Downstate Medical Center
New York University School of Medicine
St. George's University School of Medicine, Grenada, WI
USA

1. Introduction

The main aim of the chapter entitled Management Approaches to Congenital Adrenal Hyperplasia (CAH) in Adolescents and Adults; Latest Therapeutic Developments, will be first to familiarize readers with current treatment guidelines using glucocorticoid and mineralocorticoid replacement in treating this common and under-diagnosed cause of amenorrhea. Next, to introduce readers to the concept of insulin resistance in CAH and treatment approaches based upon increasing insulin sensitivity. Finally, we shall consider possible future directions in the treatment of CAH.

2. Current conventional therapy for congenital adrenal hyperplasia

2.1 Glucocorticoid replacement: Rationale, current dosing considerations and benefits

Conventional therapy for this family of disorders with glucocorticoids and sometimes mineralocorticoid remains, for now, the gold standard. The rationale for this approach is straightforward and logical. CAH is a family of disorders in which there are mutations in one or more genes for enzymes involved in adrenal (and sometimes ovarian) steroidogenesis, rendering the resultant enzyme less functional than the wild type. Alternatively, there is no mutation in the region coding for the enzyme, but one may be found, for example, in the promoter region affecting either gene expression or enzyme activity (Trapp et al., 2011).

In each of these situations the hypothalamic-pituitary-adrenal (HPA) axis goes into overdrive due to negative feed-back attempting to produce adequate levels of cortisol and sometimes aldosterone. When aldosterone synthesis is also impaired the renin-angiotensin aldosterone system (RAAS) likewise goes into overdrive (Merke & Bornstein, 2005; White, 1997).

The presence of partial blocks in the biosynthesis of cortisol and/or aldosterone results in the diversion of a portion of adrenal steroidogenesis into the available unblocked pathway, androgen synthesis. Androgen synthesis is further stimulated by the enhanced activities of the HPA and the RAAS (White, 1997).

For the most part, this strategy of providing the adrenocortical end-products, glucocorticoids and mineralocorticoids, is spectacularly successful. Instituted in the nursery this therapy will prevent severe salt wasting, dehydration and death in infants born with severe, salt-wasting forms of classical CAH. It prevents most progression of virilization and prepares the infant for corrective external genital surgery, if required. Begun early enough it will usually result in gender identity which is congruent with the child's chromosomal sex (Raff, 2004; Young & Hughes, 1990).

Treatment principles for adolescent and adult patients are quite similar to those used in treating adrenal insufficiency. Total daily maintenance doses of hydrocortisone range from 15 to 30 mg, of cortisone acetate from 12.5 to 37.5 mg and of prednisone from 3 to 5 mg. Dexamethasone is generally avoided because of difficulty of titration at low doses, long half life, resulting in overlap of daily doses, and its lack of any effect on the mineralocorticoid receptor (Speiser et al., 2010; Merke, 2008).

As with adrenal insufficiency, recommended doses for CAH have fallen by 25-35% over the past 10-15 years as better estimates of normal daily cortisol production have become available. With the adoption of lower doses of glucocorticoid it is anticipated that there will be a lower future prevalence of bone loss, hyperglycemia, capillary fragility, and other complications of long term glucocorticoid use (Speiser et al., 2010).

In adrenal insufficiency glucocorticoid is typically dosed in a way that approximates the diurnal rhythm of cortisol secretion e.g. the morning doses of hydrocortisone and cortisone acetate are about twice the evening doses; if prednisone is chosen it is usually dosed in the morning. In CAH the treatment concept is to suppress the diurnal morning surge in adrenal androgen production. Thus, the evening doses of hydrocortisone and cortisone acetate will be double of the morning dose. Prednisone is dosed at bedtime. This dosing schedule is also referred to as reverse circadian dosing. Some workers advocate dosing hydrocortisone and cortisone acetate 3 times a day citing more complete suppression of adrenal androgen synthesis, however, compliance becomes more difficult as the number of daily doses increases (Speiser et al., 2010; Newell-Price et al., 2008).

In patients with classic CAH, hydrocortisone doses may be need to be raised somewhat to suppress progesterone prior to attempting conception, such that a proliferative endometrium may develop, followed by a secretory endometrium in an orderly sequence which will allow implantation to occur. There is no contraindication to breast feeding for women on hydrocortisone or cortisone acetate replacement.

Dexamethasone treatment of mothers to prevent ambiguous external genitalia in the neonate is not recommended outside of well designed IRB-approved clinical trials.

2.2 Mineralocorticoid replacement: Rationale, current dosing considerations and benefits

In patients with severe, salt-wasting forms of classical CAH e.g. salt-wasting 21-hydroxylase deficiency and Visser-Cost syndrome mineralocorticoid replacement is essential in infants and young children as well as most adults. Some older children, adolescents, and adults can manage without supplemental mineralocorticoid if they maintain a high salt intake (Antal & Zhou, 2009). Even in some non-salt wasting forms of CAH there is, at least, mildly impaired aldosterone synthesis. It is recognized that in such patients mineralocorticoid replacement, while not essential for survival, does have a glucocorticoid sparing effect, allowing for maintenance of blood pressure, normal serum electrolytes, and general well being with somewhat lower doses of glucocorticoids, thus reducing the risk for bone loss, hyperglycemia, muscle weakness, and affective disturbances. Normalization of the plasma renin activity (PRA) may be used as a barometer for adequate mineralocorticoid replacement. Usual adult mineralocorticoid replacement is with fludrocortisones 0.05- 0.15 mg daily.

2.3 Sick day and stress dose adjustments of glucocorticoids and mineralocorticoids

Stress adjustments of glucocorticoids in CAH are similar to those in adrenal insufficiency. Mild stresses such as upper respiratory infections, minor injuries, and minor surgery require a doubling of the dose for 1-3 days. More serious stresses e.g. pneumonia, major fractures, or major surgery will require full stress doses of glucocorticoid e.g. 50-100 mg of hydrocortisone by intravenous piggyback or continuous infusion every 6-8 hours. As with daily maintenance doses of glucocorticoids for adrenal insufficiency, stress glucocorticoid dosage recommendations have fallen for CAH as well. There is now the realization that vascular tone, normalization of serum sodium, and prevention of hypoglycemia in ill and critically CAH patients can be achieved and maintained with significantly lower doses of glucocorticoid then previously prescribed. The current practice reduces the risk of inducing severe hyperglycemia, hypokalemia, and affective changes (Speiser et al., 2010). Intravenous bolus (push) doses of glucocorticoids should be avoided as they have been reported to cause dysrhythmias (Fujimoto et al., 1990).

Mineralocorticoid doses do not generally have to be increased for stress. On mild stress days patients can be instructed to increase their salt and water intake. On severe stress days the use of intravenous 5% dextrose in 0.9 normal saline at about 3 liters/day in combination with high dose hydrocortisone, which has some mineralocorticoid activity at high serum levels, and will bind as an agonist to mineralocorticoid receptors, will provide adequate electrolyte and water homeostasis. Nevertheless, if hyponatremia or hypotension persist, fludrocortisone should be initiated or its dosage should be raised. (Connery & Coursin, 2004; Riepe & Sippell, 2007). Stress glucocorticoid doses should be tapered as rapidly as the patient's precipitating condition allows, monitoring serum glucose and electrolytes as well as blood pressure carefully (Connery & Cousin, 2004).

Clearly, the treatment of the CAHs with glucocorticoids and mineralocorticoids has been one of the outstanding advances in modern medicine. It has been lifesaving for countless infants with classical CAH and has allowed for chromosomally congruent gender identification in many affected patients. It has ameliorated problems such as premature epiphysial closure with reduced adult height, hirsutism, acne, alopecia, menstrual disorders, and hypofertility/infertility. Associated polycystic ovaries often normalize their appearance on ultrasound.

2.4 Limitations of glucocorticoid and mineralocorticoid therapy

In the non-classical CAHs (NCAH), especially those with milder functional abnormalities of the affected enzyme or in some affected heterozygotes, it is often possible to normalize the production of adrenal androgens and steroid intermediates such as 17-hydroxyprogesterone, 17-hydroxypregnenolone, and 11-deoxycortisol with low replacement doses. However, in the more severely affected patients production of androgens and intermediates may remain quite high with symptomatic implications (Merke & Bornstein, 2005).

We are cautioned, appropriately, in these patients not to normalize androgen and intermediate production at the expense of treating with supraphysiologic glucocorticoid doses, which may cause bone loss, hyperglycemia, weight gain, and other more subtle features of hypercortisolism. We are left, in these patients, to treat the remaining hyperandrogenism with androgen receptor blockers, e.g. spironolactone, which also reduces ovarian/adrenal androgen production (Merke & Bornstein, 2005; Merke, 2008).

Oral contraceptives are frequently prescribed as adjunctive treatment to suppress associated ovarian hyperandrogenism and to impose a regular menstrual cycle (Merke, 2008). Recently, inhibitors of 5α-reductase, finasteride and dutasteride, have been utilized to reduce the conversion of testosterone to dihydrotestosterone, the steroid compound most directly responsible for acne, alopecia, and hirsutism. Of the two medications, dutasteride is the more effective because it inhibits both forms of the enzyme (Choi et al., 2010). Additional strategies include the use of electrolysis for permanent removal of unwanted hair, laser for semi-permanent hair removal, depilatories for temporary hair removal, cosmetic bleaching of hair, benzoyl peroxide and retinoic acid derivatives for acne control and tetracyline, and its derivatives for suppression of *Propionibacterium acnes* in acne.

3. The concept of insulin resistance in congenital adrenal hyperplasia

3.1 Similarities to and overlap with polycystic ovarian syndrome

Clinically, the features of the non-classical adrenal hyperplasias (NCAH's) are:

- premature adrenarche
- menstrual irregularity
- hypofertility/infertility
- acne
- hirsutism
- alopecia
- central adiposity
- acanthosis nigricans
- skin tags
- increased risk of Type 2 diabetes mellitus (T2DM)
- polycystic ovaries

These are nearly identical with those of polycystic ovarian syndrome (PCOS) (Pall et al., 2010). PCOS, which so closely resembles NCAH, is universally recognized to be associated with insulin resistance and is reported to be responsive to the insulin sensitizers metformin (Franks, 2011; Ladson et al., 2011) , troglitazone, rosiglitazone and pioglitazone (Franks, 2011). One report (Paoletti et al., 1996) showed that many patients with PCOS responded to the dopamine receptor agonist, cabergoline, a compound which is now used in the treatment of T2DM. Given the multitude of similarities between PCOS and NCAH it seemed reasonable to believe that NCAH patients, like PCOS patients might be insulin resistant

3.2 Possible mechanisms of insulin resistance in cah

Review of studies linking CAH with insulin resistance and those showing biochemical/phenotypic amelioration with interventions that reduce insulin resistance invites the question - by what mechanism(s) do insulin resistance/hyperinsulinemia affect the expression of CAH?

It is known that many factors affect the expression of both normal and mutant genes-the levels of transcription, translation, and post-translational gene product function. The nuclear transcription factor, peroxisome proliferator-activated receptor gamma (PPAR-γ) affects the expression of a wide variety of genes. PPAR-γ is found in both the corticotrophs of the anterior pituitary and the adrenal cortex (Mannelli et al., 2010). Short, interfering RNA's (siRNA's) can silence transcription of normal or mutant genes as reported by Inoue et al., 2006.

Hyperinsulinemia increases the biosynthesis of androgen by the adrenal cortex as reported by Arslanian et al (2002). This is partially due to an insulin-induced, post-translational hyperphosphorylation of P450c17α, resulting in an increase in its 17,20 lyase activity in both adrenals and ovaries, thus magnifying the effect of any distal, adrenal steroidogenic defect.

Kelly et al reported that steroidogenic factor-1 (SF-1) activity is upregulated in vitro by insulin in the presence of forskolin (a functional analog of ACTH) in this setting. Increased SF-1 synthesis, as well as increased binding of SF-1 to its response element, resulted in increased transcription of CYP17 causing increased adrenal androgen synthesis in both normal, human adrenocortical tissue and in cultures of the adrenocortical tumor line H-295. In these same two *in vitro* systems insulin inhibited the forskolin stimulated synthesis of the transcription factor *nur77*, an action that results in decreased transcription of CYP21 mRNA, further directing adrenal steroidogenesis toward androgen vs cortisol biosynthesis. Thus, hyperinsulinemia would worsen the phenotypic/biochemical expression of 21-hydroxylase deficiency as well as magnify any other deficiencies of adrenal steroidogenic enzymes (Kelly et al., 2004).

3.3 Review of studies demonstrating insulin resistance in congenital adrenal hyperplasia

3.3.1 Hyperandrogenemia as a general accompaniment of the insulin-resistant state, type 2 diabetes mellitus

Andersson et al. reported that women with T2DM had significantly higher plasma insulin concentrations, lower sex hormone binding globulin (SHBG), and higher circulating free testosterone levels than did BMI and gender matched controls. Men with T2DM had significantly lower total serum testosterone than a matched group of non-diabetic men, but no significant difference in their circulating free testosterone levels. They concluded that women with T2DM were relatively hyperandrogenemic and men with T2DM were normoandrogenic (Andersson et al., 1994).

We noted (Sacerdote et al., 1994, 1995) that both hyperinsulinemia and hyperandrogenemia will suppress SHBG, resulting in lower total serum testosterone in both men and women. We added that other androgens, not measured in their study, e.g. androstenedione and DHEA might be contributing to the lowering of SHBG in both sexes. We reported that all 66 of our consecutive, non-selected, type 2 diabetic patients (60 men and 6 women aged 29-89), had evidence of adrenal hyperandrogenemia as evidenced by elevated basal or cosyntropin-stimulated serum androstenedione, DHEA, DHEA-S, free testosterone, or adrenal steroid intermediates eg 17-hydroxyprogesterone. In our series, the most frequent steroid elevations were of 17-OH-progesterone and 17-OH-pregnenolone, but we also reported glucocorticoid-suppressible elevations of 11-deoxycortisol, and deoxycorticosterone (DOC). In addition, we reported glucocorticoid-reversible depressions of SHBG. Both Andersson's study (Andersson et al., 1994) and ours noted an association between hyperandrogenism and Type 2 DM-an insulin-resistant state.

3.3.2 Non-classical 21-hydroxylase deficiency

Speiser et al. reported insulin resistance in six women with untreated non-classical 21-hydroxylase deficiency using a tolbutamide-modified, frequently-sampled intravenous glucose tolerance test (Speiser et al., 1992). These findings of Speiser's were confirmed in 18 untreated women with non-classical 21-hydroxylase deficiency using the HOMA-IR (Saygili et al., 2005). Singer et al. reported persistence of insulin resistance in a patient with non-classical 21-hydroxylase deficiency after normalization of her serum androgens with glucocorticoid, indicating that the hyperandrogenism was not contributing to the insulin resistance or, alternatively, that any insulin resistance due to hyperandrogenemia was replaced by insulin resistance due to glucocorticoid (Singer et al., 1989). Kroese et al. compared 12 glucocorticoid -treated adult patients with non-classical CAH with 12 controls determining insulin sensitivity by euglycemic clamp and oral glucose tolerance testing. CAH patients were insulin resistant compared with controls. Treatment with pioglitazone 45 mg improved insulin sensitivity and lowered blood pressure in CAH patients (Kroese et al., 2009). In a study of 203 patients with CAH, 199 of whom had 21-hydroxylase deficiency, in the care of specialized endocrine centers across the United Kingdom National Health Service, it was found that 41% were obese and 29% were insulin resistant (Arit et al., 2010). Pall et al. reported that insulin sensitivity in women with non-classical 21-hydroxylase deficiency was indistinguishable from that of lean women with PCOS (Pall et al., 2010). In a meta-analysis it was concluded that NCAH was associated with increased fat mass, BMI, insulin resistance, and the metabolic syndrome (Mooij et al., 2010).

3.3.3 Classical 21-hydroxylase deficiency

Charmandari et al. reported that that, compared to children without classical CAH (n=28), children with classical 21-hydroxylase deficiency (n=16), both salt-wasters (n=12) and those with the simple virilizing phenotype (n=4) had significantly more insulin resistance as assessed by HOMA-IR as well as significantly higher serum leptin levels (Charmandari et al., 2002). Zhang et al. reported that, compared with matched controls, 30 young adult women with classical, simple virilizing 21-hydroxylase deficiency (not on glucocorticoid treatment) had significantly higher BMI, 2-hour post-load plasma glucose, serum triglycerides, fasting insulin, and HOMA-IR as well as lower serum HDL. Serum adiponectin (considered a marker for insulin sensitivity) was markedly lower in the CAH patients. Linear regression analyses revealed that higher serum testosterone concentrations were significantly, positively correlated with metabolic disorder indices and negatively correlated with serum adiponectin concentration (Zhang et al., 2010). Zimmerman et al. studied 27 patients with classical 21-hydroxylase deficiency, aged 4-31 on glucocorticoid replacement and a like number of sex, age, and BMI matched controls. They found that LDL, fasting serum glucose, insulin, and HOMA-IR were significantly higher in the patients with classical 21-hydroxylase deficiency, while HDL was significantly lower. These authors attributed the adverse metabolic changes to glucocorticoid therapy as HOMA-IR showed a significant positive correlation with hydrocortisone dose (Zimmerman et al., 2010). Atabek et al. reported a 5 year old girl with female pseudohermaphroditism due to classical 21-hydroxylase deficiency with insulin resistance and Turner's syndrome. These authors noted an improvement in insulin sensitivity when their patient was treated for hyperandrogenemia with glucocorticoid (Atabek et al., 2005). Ambroziak et al. reported that adult patients with classical 21-hydroxylase deficiency have obesity, hyperinsulinemia, insulin resistance, and hyperleptinemia more frequently than age/sex matched controls (Ambroziak et al., 2010).

3.3.4 Non-classical 3-β-ol dehydrogenase deficiency

Carbunaru et al. have reported that the hormonal phenotype of non-classic 3-β-ol dehydrogenase deficiency in hyperandrogenemic females is associated with insulin-resistant

PCOS and is not a variant of genetic HSD3B2 deficiency (Carbunaru et al., 2004). This article is consistent with a publication by (Lutfallah et al., 2002) that proposed new hormonal criteria for the diagnosis of those patients with mutations in the Type II 3-beta-ol dehydrogenase exon. They noted that in the vast majority of patients who had been diagnosed with non-classic 3-β-ol dehydrogenase deficiency using criteria analogous to those used to diagnose non-classic 21-hydroxylase deficiency no mutation could be found in the HSD3B exon. This, of course, does not exclude the possibility that these patients could harbor mutations in the extra-exonic portions of the gene, for example in the promoter region, as has recently been reported in some patients with 21-hydroxylase deficiency (Araújo et al., 2007). In addition, other factors may affect the transcription, translation, or post-translation activity of steroidogenic genes. For example, insulin up-regulates the transcription of 17-α-hydroxylase and downregulates the transcription of 21-hydroxylase (Kelly et al., 2004), while it also causes a post-translational hyperphosphorylation of P450c17α resulting in a gain of function in its 17,20 lyase activity in both the ovaries and the adrenal cortex which, in turn, magnifies the effects of any distal adrenal steroidogenic enzyme defects and potentiates the effect of LH on ovarian androgen synthesis (Arslanian et al., 2002). Genes with perfectly normal nucleotide sequences may have their transcription blocked by excessive methylation or aberrant histone acetylation.

3.3.5 Other forms of non-classical CAH associated with insulin resistance

Our reports on adrenal hyperandrogenemia and T2DM (Sacerdote et al., 1994, 1995) clearly included patients with 3-β-ol dehydrogenase deficiency and aldosterone synthase deficiency and some who were not definitively characterized, but who had glucocorticoid-suppressible elevations of androstenedione, DHEA, DHEA-S, and free/total serum testosterone as well as glucocrticoid normalizable depressions of SHBG. In Arit's study four of 203 patients with CAH had forms of NCAH other than 21-hydroxylase deficiency (Arit et al., 2010). We studied 26 consecutive, non-selected psychiatric patients taking classical anti-psychotic agents, atypical anti-psychotic agents, and/or valproate and we noted that all 26 had adrenal hyperandrogenemia; 2 had biochemical evidence of 21-hydroxylase deficiency, 8 of 3-β-ol–dehydrogenase deficiency, four of 11-hydroxylase deficiency, and two of aldosterone synthase deficiency (Bahtiyar et al., 2007). All of the above psychotropic agents cause insulin resistance and 10/10 patients who took an insulin sensitizer normalized biochemically.

3.3.6 Studies linking insulin resistance with forms of classical CAH other than 21-hydroxylase deficiency

Charmandari et al.'s series reporting elevated serum leptin levels and insulin resistance in children with classic CAH included 2 patients with 11-hydroxylase deficiency (Charmandari et al., 2002).

4. Studies showing utility of insulin sensitization in adrenal hyperplasia

4.1 Metformin and/or thiazolidinediones in the non-classical adrenal hyperplasias

In 2000 we reported that metformin alone or, in some patients, with the first thiazolidinedione (TZD) troglitazone, normalized elevated serum steroid metabolites and ameliorated acne, alopecia, and hirsutism in patients with T2DM and non-classical forms of 21-hydroxylase deficiency, 11-hydroxylase deficiency, 3-β-ol dehydrogenase deficiency, and aldosterone synthase deficiency (Osehobo et al., 2000). In 2003 we reported that the biochemical /phenotypic expression of NCAH, including 21-hydroxylase deficiency, 3-β-ol dehydrogenase deficiency, 11-hydroxylase deficiency, and aldosterone synthase deficiency could be normalized with rosiglitazone, an example of which may be seen in (Sacerdote et al., 2003) [Figure 1]. In 2004 we reported that the biochemical/phenotypic expression of NCAH is correctible with pioglitazone (Sacerdote et al., 2004). An example of the combined effect of metformin and pioglitazone as compared with standard treatment in a patient with non-classical 21-hydroxylase deficiency is shown in Figure 2. Note that the suppression of 17-OH-progesterone is more complete with the combined insulin sensitizers and even with metformin

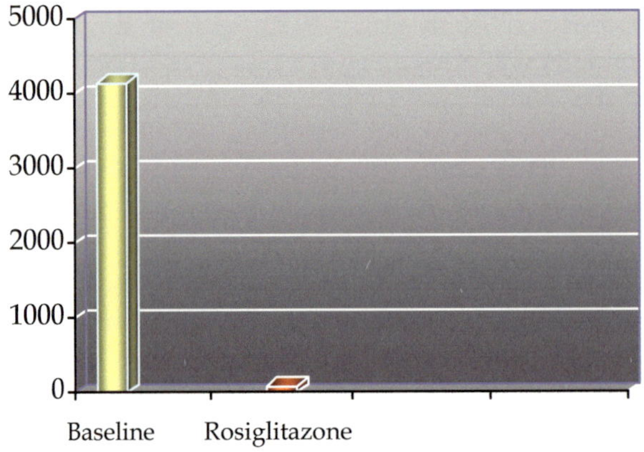

Fig. 1. Response of a 43-year-old Male's 17-OHP (ng/dl) to rosiglitazone 4mg twice daily.

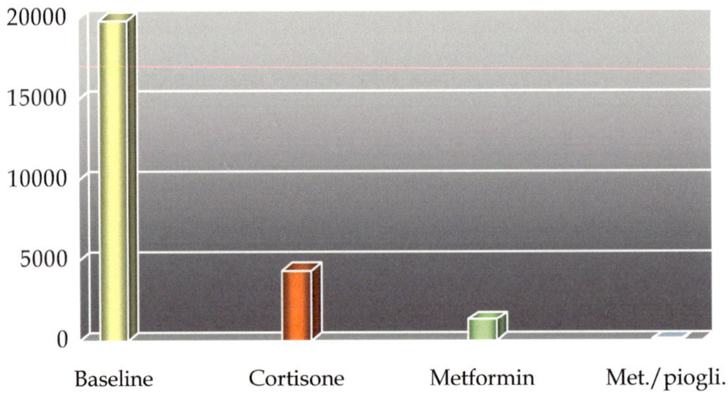

Fig. 2. Response of a 57-year-old Female's 17-OHP (ng/dl) to cortisone acetate, metformin, & pioglitazone

monotherapy than it is with standard treatment. Arslanian et al. reported that metformin treatment in obese teens with PCOS and impaired glucose tolerance (IGT) ameliorated their exaggerated adrenal response to ACTH with concomitant reduction in insulinemia/insulin resistance (Arslanian et al., 2002). The time course of biochemical improvement in NCAH patients treated with metformin or a TZD is quite rapid-within 24 hours of initiating therapy.

4.1.2 Metformin or rosiglitazone in the psychotropic/valproate-induced adrenal hyperplasias

Many medications exert an endocrine disrupter effect by virtue of directly causing insulin resistance or indirectly causing insulin resistance by increasing appetite with resultant weight gain. Among these are both classical and atypical anti-psychotic drugs, valproate, which has also been associated with PCOS (Bilo & Meo, 2008), nucleoside analogs, and protease inhibitors. The latter two groups of anti-retroviral drugs have also been associated with adrenal hyperplasia (Sacerdote, 2006). In our study we found that metformin corrected adrenal hyperandrogenism in 8/8 patients and rosiglitazone corrected adrenal hyperandrogenism in 2/2 patients on anti-psychotic drugs and/or valproate (Bahtiyar, 2007). (Figures 3 and 4).

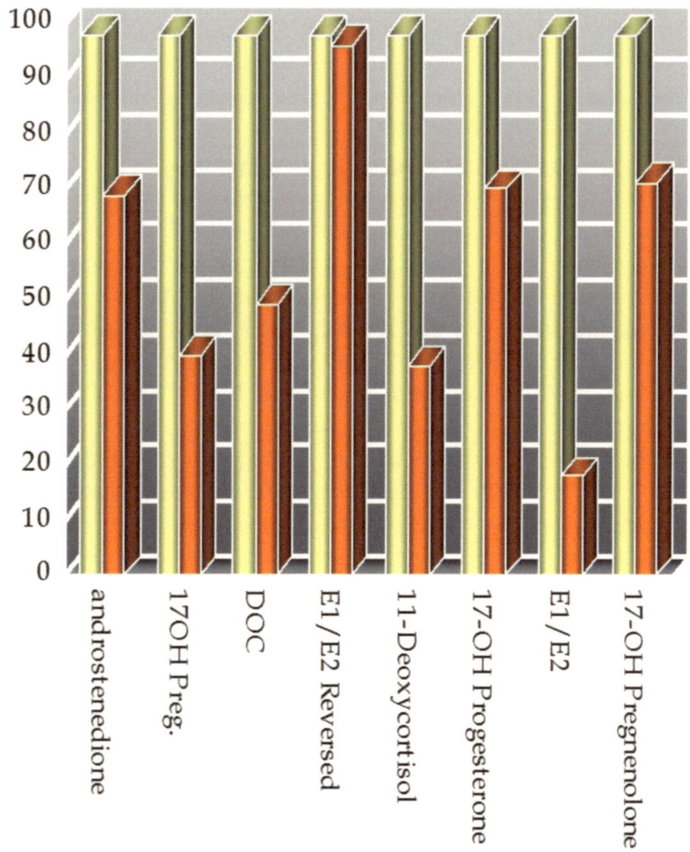

Fig. 3. Effect of metformin on elevated steroid metabolites (Represented a % of baseline). lightly shaded bars are baselines; darkly shaded bars are on metformin treatment.

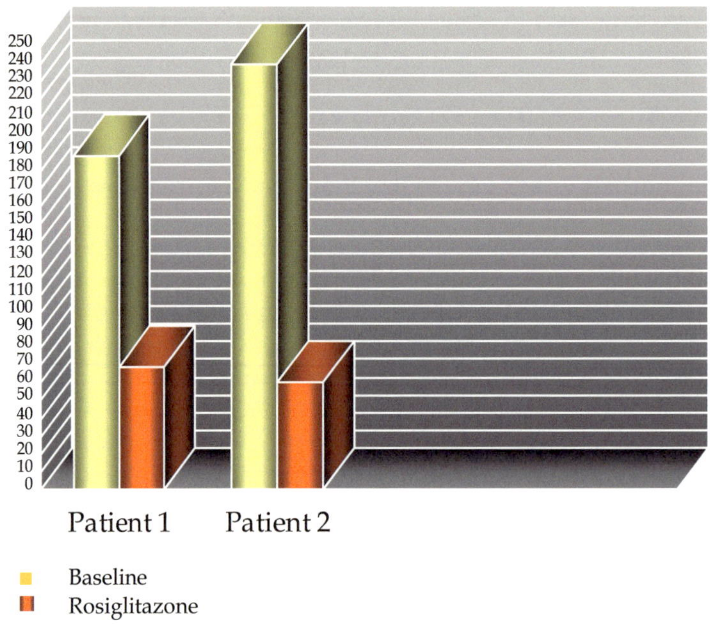

Fig. 4. Effect of rosiglitazone on elevated baseline 11-deoxycortisol level (mg/dl)

4.1.3 Metformin to treat classical 21-hydroxylase deficiency

Because the classical CAH's are much less common than the non-classical forms and also because we are adult endocrinologists and many adolescent/adult classical CAH patients tend to remain in the care of their pediatric endocrinologists, it was a number of years from when we first conceived the notion of treating classical CAH with insulin sensitizers until we were able to participate in the treatment of a classical CAH patient through the collaboration of a pediatric endocrine colleague, Dr. Levon Agdere (Mapas-Dimaya et al, 2008). Our patient was a 17-year-old female who was born with ambiguous genitalia and developed severe hyponatremia and dehydration in the nursery, where she was correctly diagnosed and appropriately treated. At one year of age she underwent clitoroplasty. During 4 years of treatment with her previous pediatric endocrinologist her vital signs and electrolytes remained normal and her height was 142.33 cm which was below the third percentile for her age. A bone age performed at 15.5 years was slightly advanced at 16.0 years. Since age 13 she had been on hydrocortisone 30 mg/day given in two divided reverse circadian doses (10 mg in am and 20 mg in pm) as well as fludrocortisones 0.05 mg daily. Medication compliance was verified with pill counts and refill data. On this regimen she continued to have normal serum electrolytes, glucose, blood pressure, and external genitals, but she noted truncal obesity, hirsutism, acanthosis nigricans, and amenorrhea. Her 17-OH-progesterone remained persistently elevated at 3410 ng/dl (20-500) as was her serum total testosterone at 326 ng/dl (15-70). She was maintained on her glucocorticoid/ mineralocorticoid regime and after obtaining the informed consent of the patient and her parents metformin 500 mg orally after breakfast and supper was added. As seen in Figures 5 and 6 both steroid metabolites fell by about 50% on this combined regimen to 1539 ng/dl and 163 ng/dl respectively. Her amenorrhea resolved and her hirsutism improved. Our long term intention was to gradually up-titrate her metformin dose and, if necessary, add a TZD until levels of both steroid metabolites normalized and then begin a cautious tapering of her glucocorticoid dosage, however, our patient declared herself satisfied with her initial improvement and declined to undergo further adjustments in her treatment or further testing.

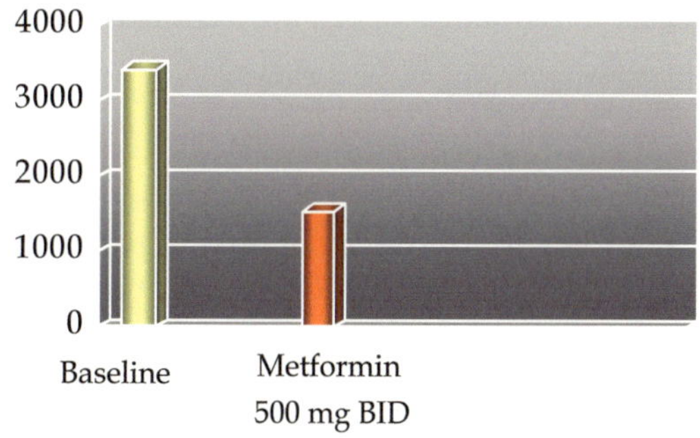

Fig. 5. Effect of metformin addition on 17-OHP (ng/dl) in a patient with classical, salt-wasting 21-hydroxylase deficiency

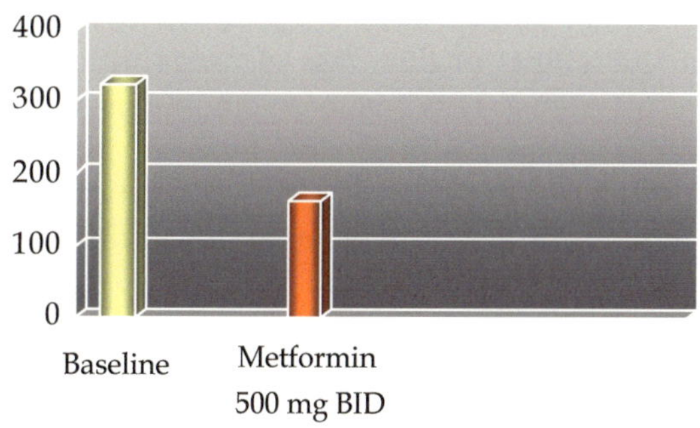

Fig. 6. Effect of metformin on serum total testosterone (ng/dl) in classical 21-hydroxylase deficiency

4.1.4 Limitations of metformin and thiazolidinediones in the treatment of CAH

Although metformin has been shown to be effective as monotherapy or with a TZD for several forms of NCAH and as an adjunctive therapy for classical, salt-losing 21-hydroxylase deficiency, it is currently unknown whether metformin would be an effective treatment for classical, simple virilizing 21-hydroxylase deficiency or for any other form of classical CAH. We do not know if metformin monotherapy or combination therapy with a TZD could ultimately replace glucocorticoid completely in any of the classical CAH's.

In women with PCOS, metformin has been shown, not only to be safe to use throughout pregnancy, but to reduce hyperinsulinemia, weight gain, gestational diabetes mellitus (GDM), and spontaneous abortion (Glueck et al., 2004; Jakubowicz et al., 2002). Metformin is generally considered safe in both gestational and pre-gestational diabetes mellitus and GDM as it is U.S. F.D.A. Class B. There is also evidence that is safe in nursing mothers (Feig et al., 2007).

Many patients are unable to tolerate the gastrointestinal side effects of metformin, particularly at maximally effective doses. The tolerability of metformin may be increased by a number of different strategies:

- Administration after meals
- Gradual dose titration to allow for adaptation to the drug
- Use of extended release preparations which are better tolerated than the short acting tablets
- Use of liquid preparations (Riomet^R)
- Use of extended release polymer form (Glumetza^R)
- Addition of an H_2 blocker or proton pump inhibitor

Metformin should be avoided or very closely monitored in patients with Stage III or worse chronic kidney disease, patients with serious bacterial infections, and for at least two days before and after administration of iodinated intravenous radiographic contrast materials or before and after major surgery, so as not to increase the risk of lactic acidosis. There is little risk of serious hypoglycemia with metformin monotherapy, but mild hypoglycemia may occur if meals are skipped, skimped, or delayed. Serum vitamin B12 and folate levels should be checked periodically in patients using metformin as deficiencies may develop resulting in elevated serum homocysteine levels and peripheral neuropathy, especially in patients with comorbid diabetes.

TZD's have been shown to ameliorate the biochemical/phenotypic findings in most forms of NCAH. To date there are no studies or case reports where they have been used to treat classic CAH. Common side effects of this class of drugs include weight gain, increased subcutaneous fat mass, and edema. Less common, but more serious adverse effects of this class include: congestive heart failure, bone loss, fracture, and bladder carcinoma. With regard to the latter, we have unpublished data in one diabetic patient suggesting reversibility of pre-macroscopic bladder carcinoma after withdrawal of TZD's.

TZD-mediated edema appears to respond well to thiazides, spironolactone, triamterene, and, in our experience, to the renin antagonist aliskerin. It is somewhat resistant to loop diuretics such as furosemide. Data from the PROactive study (Dormandy J et al, 2009) indicate that congestive heart failure developing in patients taking TZD's is no more treatment refractory or lethal than that occurring in Type 2 diabetic patients not using TZD's.

To date there are no randomized control trials (RCT's) on treatment or prevention of TZD-associated bone loss, although in the authors' experience osteopenic/osteoporotic TZD users respond satisfactorily to standard treatments.

The use of rosiglitazone in the treatment of T2DM has been questioned as a result of a meta-analysis published by Nissen and Wolski (Nissen & Wolski, 2007) reporting a "signal" of increased risk of myocardial infarction in rosiglitazone users compared to Type 2 diabetics not using this drug. This report, while controversial, has resulted in rosiglitazone being banned in the EU and severely restricted in the US.

Although many women have become pregnant while taking TZD's either for T2DM or for PCOS and there have not been reports of an adverse effect upon the pregnancies, there have been no published reports of their use beyond the first trimester. It is recommended that TZD's be stopped when pregnancy is suspected or confirmed. TZD monotherapy does not result in hypoglycemia.

5. Utility of lifestyle interventions in the treatment of non-classic aldosterone synthase deficiency

We first reported the non-classic form of aldosterone synthase deficiency in 1999 (Osehobo & Sacerdote, 1999). Before this only the rare, severe salt-wasting form of this disorder (Visser-Cost syndrome) was known. Subsequently we reported that the biochemical/phenotypic expression of non-classic aldosterone synthase deficiency could be normalized by weight loss and exercise, two interventions that reduce insulin resistance in two women with this disorder (Sacerdote, 2002). (Figure 7).

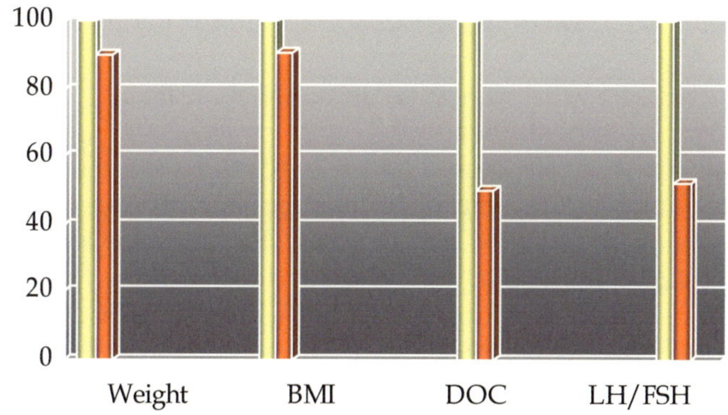

Fig. 7. Percent changes with weight loss and exercise in two women with non-classic aldosterone synthase deficiency. Light bars are baselines, shaded bars are post-treatment

6. Utility of gastric bypass surgery in the treatment of non-classical 11-hydroxylase deficiency

Recently we found that a patient of ours with non-classical 11-hydroxylase deficiency, T2DM, and morbid obesity who underwent Roux en Y gastric bypass surgery normalized her serum 11-deoxycortisol as effectively with surgery as she previously had done with metformin plus pioglitazone (Figure 8). Roux-en-Y gastric bypass has previously been reported to ameliorate PCOS (Eid et al., 2005).

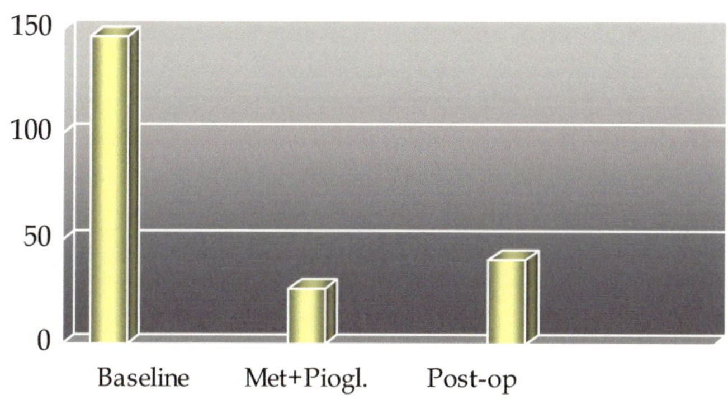

Fig. 8. Response of Patient's 11-deoxycortisol (ng/dl) to Roux-en-Y Gastric Bypass. (Normal < 51)

7. Future directions

7.1 Large randomized control trials of metformin/thiazolidinediones in classical CAH

While the therapeutic efficacy of metformin and TZD's in NCAH is fairly well established, we only have a single case report of metformin being used in classical CAH. We do not know whether metformin and/or TZD's can completely normalize serum levels of 17-hydroxyprogesterone and testosterone when added to steroid "replacement" , nor is it yet known whether metformin/TZD could actually render steroid replacement unnecessary in treating classical salt-wasting 21-hydroxylase deficiency. We have no data as to whether these insulin sensitizers have any efficacy in the treatment of any other form of classical CAH. Well designed RCT's will be necessary to answer these important questions.

7.2 Other insulin sensitizers in congenital adrenal hyperplasia

7.2.1 Dopamine agonist pilot studies

Increasing dopaminergic tone has been reported to have an insulin sensitizing effect (Pijl et al., 2000; Scranton R et al., 2010) and dopamine receptor agonists e.g. bromocriptine are approved for the treatment of T2DM and PCOS, while dopamine receptor antagonists are known to be associated with insulin` resistance and increase the risk for development of glucose intolerance. Cabergoline is used successfully in treating PCOS (Paoletti et al., 1996) as is bromocriptine (Spruce et al., 1984). On this basis we might predict that CAH might improve if treated with dopamine agonists.

7.2.2 Vitamin D pilot studies

Studies in animals show that vitamin D deficiency is associated with impaired insulin sensitivity, and that insulin secretion can be increased by vitamin D supplementation (Tai et al., 2008). Epidemiological studies in man show associations between low vitamin D levels and glucose intolerance (Nunlee et al., 2011). Pittas et al. systematically reviewed the intervention trial evidence for the role of vitamin D and/or calcium in the prevention of metabolic syndrome and T2DM (Pittas et al., 2007). On the basis of evidence from small intervention trials or post hoc analyses of trials, they concluded that it was difficult to be definite whether or not vitamin D and/or calcium were important in the prevention of T2DM, and that effects might only be manifest in people who were particularly at risk of T2DM. Other authors have implicated Vitamin D deficiency/insufficiency in the pathogenesis of insulin resistance, pre-diabetes, T2DM, and PCOS (Cavalier et al., 2011; Wehr et al., 2011). Rashidi et al reported that supplementation of just 400 IU daily of Vitamin D increased the ovulation rate significantly when added to 1500 mg/day of metformin (Rashidi et al., 2009). We have just begun to collect Vitamin D data on some of our NCAH patients and the first three have 25-OH-Vitamin D levels ranging from 18-19 ng /dl. These include one patient with 21-hydroxylase deficiency, 1 with p450-oxidoreductase deficiency, and one male patient with glucocorticoid-suppressible elevated DHEA-S. Given this data it may be reasonable to embark on pilot studies utilizing Vitamin D as monotherapy or in combination with other agents in the treatment of NCAH.

7.2.3 Bile acid binding pilot studies

The bile acid binding resin, colesevelam, has recently been approved for the treatment of T2DM in addition to its original indication for the treatment of hypercholesterolemia. It improves insulin resistance in a diet-induced rodent model by increasing the release of GLP-

1 (Zhang et al., 2010). In a pilot study Schwartz et al. reported that in patients with T2DM colesevelam had no effect on peripheral insulin sensitivity or glucose absorption, but may improve glycemic control by improving whole body insulin sensitivity. Pilot studies with this agent in both PCOS and NCAH might be warranted due to its insulin sensitizing effects (Schwartz et al., 2010).

7.2.4 GLP-1 agonist pilot studies

The GLP-1 agonists exenatide and liraglutide are both associated with weight loss, the latter somewhat more so. The weight loss, particularly that of visceral and non-adipose tissue fat, is associated with an improvement in insulin sensitivity (Liu et al., 2010; Defronzo et al., 2010). Exenatide has been reported to ameliorate PCOS (Elkind-Hirsch et al., 2008). Therefore, it seems reasonable to plan pilot studies with these agents in CAH.

7.2.5 Orlistat pilot studies

The fat absorption blocking agent orlistat is approved as a weight loss aid when combined with diet and exercise in the U.S. in both a 60 gm over the counter form and a prescription only 120 mg form. In Canada it is approved for the treatment of T2DM. Panidis et al. reported that orlistat in combination with diet produced significant weight loss and improvement in insulin sensitivity in obese women, with or without PCOS. In addition, serum testosterone levels were significantly improved in women with PCOS (Panidis et al., 2008). Based on these data pilot studies of orlistat in NCAH should be performed.

7.2.6 Cannabinoid receptor blockade pilot studies

Stimulation of the CB-1 cannabinoid receptor has known orexic and euphoric effects, while its blockade with rimonabant has been associated with anorexic and dysphoric effects and results in weight loss, reduced insulin resistance, and improvements in glycemia and serum lipid levels (Migrenne et al., 2009) and has shown efficacy in PCOS patients (Sathyapalan et al., 2008). Rimonabant was not approved in the U.S. and its approval was withdrawn in Europe because of a higher suicide risk due, presumably, to its dysphoric effect. The risk/benefit ratio of this class of agents might be improved by better patient selection, selective co-administration of an anti-depressant, treatment of hyperhomocysteinemia (which may play a role in depression, or the development of selective cannabinoid receptor modulators, possessing the beneficial anorexic effect of the class without causing dysphoria. The selective estrogen receptor modulators (SERM's), now in widespread clinical use, provide a model for such future development. Since these agents reduce insulin resistance, we might predict that they could ameliorate CAH.

7.2.7 Continuous positive airway pressure (CPAP) in CAH patients with obstructive sleep apnea (OSA)

Many, if not most, insulin resistant people have OSA (Vgontzas et al., 2005). Treatment with CPAP has been shown to improve insulin sensitivity in women with PCOS (Tasali et al., 2011). Vgontzas et al have reported that the inflammatory cytokines, TNF-α and IL-6 are elevated in patients with OSA, independently of obesity and that visceral fat was the primary parameter linked with OSA (Vgontzas et al., 2005). The fact that they found that OSA was more common in women with PCOS suggested a pathogenetic role of insulin resistance in OSA. The beneficial effect of a cytokine antagonist on excessive daytime sleepiness in obese, male apneics and on sleep disordered breathing in a general, random sample supports the hypothesis that cytokines and associated insulin resistance are mediators of excessive daytime sleepiness and OSA. Hamada et al have reported that with nasal CPAP in a CAH patient with OSA they were able to reduce the maintenance glucocorticoid dosage (Hamada et al., **2011**). CAH patients who have clinical features consistent with OSA, might benefit from undergoing a sleep study followed by a CPAP titration study if the initial sleep study is diagnostic. Alternatively, inhibitors of TNF-α and IL-6 might be useful adjuncts in the treatment of CAH.

7.2.8 Curcumin

Curcumin is a component of the popular spice, turmeric. It has been reported to decrease levels of the inflammatory cytokine, TNF-α, which, in turn, downregulates the transcription factor PPAR-γ. Administration of curcumin results in up-regulation of PPAR-γ m-RNA and protein, which we would predict would improve insulin sensitivity (Gosh et al., 2009). Pilot studies with curcumin in CAH patients, would, therefore, be of interest given the absence of any known adverse effects. Other spices, herbs, and supplements known or suspected to have insulin sensitizing effects would also be worth exploring in CAH.

7.2.9 L-carnitine

L-carnitine has been reported to reduce insulin resistance, when added to orlistat, significantly more than orlistat alone (Derosa et al., 2010). For this reason, a pilot study treating CAH patients with this supplement would be of value.

7.3 Other insulin-lowering agents

7.3.1 Somatostatin analogs

Somatostatin and its analogs- octreotide, octreotide LAR, and lanreotide partially suppress insulin secretion; reduction of hyperinsulinemia by this means could result in amelioration of both PCOS and CAH. Gambineri's group reported that octreotide-LAR improved the ovulation rate and hirsutism and showed nearly significant trends toward greater reductions in serum testosterone and androstenedione compared with placebo in dieting women with abdominal obesity and PCOS (Gambineri et al., 2005). Pilot studies of these drugs in these two conditions, would, therefore, be of interest. Because they reduce the secretion of growth hormone they would not be suitable for use in children or adolescents.

7.3.2 Diazoxide and phenytoin

These drugs both decrease insulin secretion and have been reported to be helpful in treating some PCOS patients (Bercovici et al., 1996; Verrotti et al., 2011). On this basis we might predict a response in CAH patients as well. In designing pilot studies with these agents patients with pre-diabetes or low bone density should probably be excluded due to the diabetogenic potential of both drugs and the accelerated Vitamin D clearance attributed to the latter.

7.4 Gene therapy

Gene therapy, wherein the defective gene is supplemented with a functional one should, theoretically, be the ideal therapy for every form of CAH, with the possible exception of non-classical 3-β-ol dehydrogenase deficiency, for which no mutation in the exon has been identified (Carbunaru et al., 2004).

7.4.1 Adenoviruses

Adenoviruses are adrenocorticotropic, making them a good vector in which to deliver functional genes. 21-hydroxylase genes have been delivered in adenoviruses by intra-adrenal injection in 21-hydroxylase-deficient mice and bovine adrenocortical cells have shown functional and morphological changes in the adrenal cortices after transfection with recombinant adenovirus (Loechner et al., 2010). While encouraging, overall safety and specificity in targeting the adrenal cortex remains to be established. There may be a need to develop new vectors (viral or non-viral) to optimize the specificity and efficiency of adrenal gene transfer and ensure long term DNA integration. Recently, other recombinant viruses, e.g. retrovirus, lentivirus, adeno-associated virus, and Herpes simplex have been successfully used as gene vectors. Non-viral gene delivery methods that use natural or synthetic compounds or physical forces to deliver DNA to the cell are now available.

7.4.2 Adult stem cells

Adult stem cells may be obtained from a variety of tissues and have been studied in several milieus, especially the hematopoietic system. Limiting factors with adult stem cells include:

- Limited pluripotency
- Difficulty of maintenance in vitro
- HLA compatibility restraints on transplantation, thus requiring immunosuppression with its attendant risks, cost, and inconvenience

Recent studies have described methods which are generally applicable for the preparation of induced pluripotent stem cells (IPSC's) from various somatic cell lineages. Marrow-derived mesenchymal cells (MSC's) are unique in that they are obtained from adults, yet are still pluripotent. MSC's or IPSC's obtained from CAH patients would harbor a genetic defect in steroidogenesis and, thus, would only be helpful as cellular vectors for gene therapy. Despite their shortcomings, the use of adult stem cells benefits from a longer investigational track record and avoids ongoing political issues with the use of fetal stem cells. Yazawa et al. have reported that human MSC's transfected with SF-1, a transcription factor required for both adrenal and gonadal steroidogenesis, differentiate into cortisol producing cells rather than androgen producing cells when transplanted into mouse testis, while Gondo et al reported that such cells were ACTH-responsive (Yazawa et al., 2006; Gondo et al., 2004). Another approach is that of Hammer et al who characterized a subpopulation of adrenal cells that are typically dormant or undifferentiated. Stimulation of these cells to differentiate into mature adrenal cells is possible and studies aimed at collecting this quiescent population for differentiation/regeneration of adrenal tissue could be helpful in both CAH and adrenal insufficiency (Kim et al., 2007).

7.4.3 Embryonic stem cells

Embryonic stem cells (ESC's) offer an approach that avoids many of the problems inherent with the use of adult stem cells. ESC's harvested during the blastocyst stage are easier to culture *in vitro* and remain for longer periods in the pluripotent stage. ESC's could be triggered to differentiate into regulated, steroidogenic cells using methodologies derived from adult stem cell studies. As with adult tissue transplants, HLA matching is needed and there is the potential for graft rejection and, therefore, the necessity of using immunosuppressive therapy. The next generation of ESC's could be so closely matched that post-transplantation immunosuppressive treatment would not be needed (Loechner et al., 2010).

7.5 Corticotropin releasing hormone (CRH) antagonists

Inhibition of CRH should dampen the secretion of ACTH, which should facilitate the normalization of adrenal androgen secretion with lower doses of glucocorticoid. Pre-clinical studies with the CRH antagonist alarmin demonstrated blockage of CRH-1 receptor-induced increases, both in adrenal size and behavioral responses. CRH analogs with more extended action e.g. astressin inhibit ACTH release. CRH 9-41 reduces stress measures in sheep. Human CRH receptor antagonist trials demonstrated a reduction in CRH-associated signs of anxiety and depression. Since these studies have not unequivocally demonstrated reductions in CRH-induced ACTH secretion or an effect on cortisol secretion, their clinical relevance remains uncertain at present (Loechner et al., 2010).

7.6 Inhibition of ACTH secretion/action

The discovery of selective melanocortin receptor subtypes, eg MC2-R, for ACTH in the adrenal cortex affords the possibility of inhibition of ACTH action in the adrenal cortex with a diminution in adrenal androgen production. This approach could have a glucocorticoid sparing effect. Clinical trials will be important to assess the resilience of HPA reserve and the safety of this approach.

Blockade of ACTH secretion is under investigation. *In vitro* studies showed that ACTH release from corticotrophs is coupled with the dihydropyridine-sensitive subclass of voltage-dependent calcium channels Clinical trials in Cushing disease reported acute decreases in ACTH levels with calcium channel blockers such as nifedipine and amlodipine. A small trial reported similar magnitude plasma ACTH reductions in 13 children with either classic salt-wasting or simple, virilizing 21-hydroxylase deficiency.

Other agents which may decrease ACTH secretion include the serotonin receptor blocker, cyproheptadine, the dopamine receptor agonist, cabergoline, and the GABA receptor inhibitor, valproate. These agents have been reported to be efficacious in both Cushing disease and Nelson's syndrome, and for this reason, may prove to be helpful in CAH (Loechner et al., 2010).

7.7 Newer glucocorticoid delivery strategies

Studies of circadian cortisol delivery using either hydrocortisone infusions or modified release oral formulations demonstrate that these systems can better mimic physiologic cortisol rhythm, resulting in better glucocorticoid replacement and ACTH suppression in CAH patients. Continuous subcutaneous cortisol infusion (CSCI) has proven effective and well tolerated for over 4 years in a 14 year old CAH patient and resulted in a 50% reduction in daily cortisol dosage within the first 3 months of treatment (Loechner et al., 2010). Two glucocorticoid formulations that exploit the pharmacokinetic peak of once/day, dual-timed cortisol to mimic the diurnal variation peak of ACTH, facilitating more physiologic delivery of cortisol are currently being evaluated. *Chronocort*, one such preparation, seems promising. In a head to head study with *Cortef* dosed 3 times/day with a larger evening dose, it was reported that the *Cortef* regimen resulted in 3 distinct peaks, while a single daily peak at 0600 was noted with bedtime dosing of *Chronocort*. At 0600 levels of 17-OH-progesterone, ACTH, and androstenedione were lower with *Chronocort*, however, afternoon androgen control was better with *Cortef*.

7.8 Aromatase inhibitors

These agents will help block the conversion of androgens to estrogens and thus help block premature epiphysial closure in children and adolescents with CAH (Loechner et al., 2010).

7.9 GnRH agonists with or without growth hormone

As with central precocious puberty, GnRH agonist monotherapy or in combination with GH has been reported to improve the chances of reaching predicted adult height (PAH) in CAH patients with early puberty due to early maturation of the hypothalamic-pituitary-gonadal (HPG) axis. While GnRH agonists prevent premature epiphyseal closure, GH can prevent the stalling in vertical growth velocity that occurs otherwise when precocious puberty is either prevented or aborted (Loechner et al., 2010).

8. Summary/conclusions

In summary, a role for insulin resistance in the pathogenesis of NCAH may be suspected because of numerous similarities in the clinical expression of PCOS and NCAH.
Confirmation of the presence of insulin resistance in CAH has been reported for:

- Non-classical 21-hydroxylase deficiency
- Non-classical 3-β-ol dehydrogenase deficiency
- Non-classical 11-hydroxylase deficiency
- Classical simple virilizing 21-hydroxylase deficiency
- Classical salt-wasting 21-hydroxylase deficiency
- Classical 11-hydroxylase deficiency

Metformin, troglitazone, rosiglitazone, and pioglitazone-all agents known to reduce insulin resistance and ameliorate PCOS have been shown to phenotypically/biochemically ameliorate:

- Non-classical 21-hydroxylase deficiency
- Non-classical 3-β-ol dehydrogenase deficiency
- Non-classical 11-hydroxylase deficiency
- Non-classical aldosterone synthase deficiency
- Classical salt-wasting 21-hydroxylase deficiency

Weight loss by lifestyle modification (diet + exercise) has been shown to normalize DOC levels, the LH/FSH ratio and phenotypically ameliorate non-classical aldosterone synthase deficiency. Roux-en-Y gastric bypass has been shown to phenotypically/biochemically ameliorate non-classical 11-hydroxylase deficiency.
ALL INSULIN SENSITIZING INTERVENTIONS THUS FAR INVESTIGATED AMELIORATE EVERY FORM OF CAH TESTED TO DATE.

- While glucocorticoid/mineralocorticoid replacement/suppression has been spectacularly successful in the treatment of CAH and remains, for now, the gold standard for therapy of this family of disorders, there remain many patients for whom the goal of adequate androgen suppression, while avoiding the pitfalls of hypercortisolemia, remain elusive. Androgen receptor or 5-α-reductase blockade may be added to blunt the clinical effects of inadequately suppressed adrenal androgen secretion. In the future glucocorticoid/ mineralocorticoid therapy may be further refined by the use of novel long acting and dual peak preparations of hydrocortisone and newer steroid delivery systems e.g. CSCI. Adrenal androgen secretion may be further reduced in the future by means of CRH or ACTH blockade, while the combination of GnRH agonists with GH may help to more nearly achieve PAH.

- The recognition that insulin resistance/hyperinsulinemia is a regular feature in CAH that contributes to its biochemical/phenotypic expression has led to the finding that metformin and/or TZD's may replace standard therapy in NCAH and that metformin may be used, at least as adjunctive therapy, in classic, salt-wasting 21-hydroxylase deficiency. Exercise and weight loss have been shown to ameliorate non-classic aldosterone synthase deficiency, while Roux-en-Y gastric bypass can normalize the biochemical expression of non-classic 11-hydroxylase deficiency. Other therapies that decrease insulin levels, including those that have already shown efficacy in PCOS, seem likely to show therapeutic benefit in CAH.
- In the future it is likely that there will be further refinements in steroid replacement/suppression, more widespread use of treatments to decrease hyperinsulinemia, and further progress in gene therapy.

9. Acknowledgments

The authors thank Drs. L. Agdere and A. Mapas-Dimaya for their valuable collaboration.

10. References

Ambroziak, U.; Bednarczuk, T.; Ginalska-Malinowska, M.; Malunowicz, EM.; Grezhocińska, B.; Kamínski, P.; Bablok, L.; Przedlacki Bar-Andziak, E. (2010). Congenital adrenal hyperplasia due to 21-hydroxylase deficiency-management in adults. *Endokrynol Pol.* Vol.61, No.1, pp. 142-155

Andersson, B.; Marin, B.; Lissner, L.; Vermeulen, A.; Björntorp, P. (1994). Testosterone concentrations in women and men with NIDDM. *Diabetes Care,* Vol.17, No.5, pp. 405-411

Antal, Z.; Zhou, P. (2009). Congenital Adrenal Hyperplasia: Diagnosis, Evaluation, and Management. *Pediatr. Rev.* Vol.30, pp. e49 - e57

Atabek, ME.; Kurtoğlu, S.; Keskin, M. (2005). Female pseudohermaphroditism due to classical 21-hydroxylase deficiency and insulin resistance in a girl with Turner syndrome. *Turk Pediatr.* Vol.47, No.2, pp. 176-179

Araújo, RS.; Mendonca, BB.; Barbosa, AS.; Lin, CJ.; Marcondes, JA.; Billerbeck, AE.; Bachega, TA. (2007). Microconversion between CYP21A2 and CYP21A1P promoter regions causes the nonclassical form of 21-hydroxylase deficiency. *J Clin Endocrinol Metab.* Vol.92, No.10, pp. 4028-4034

Arit, W.; Willis, DS.; Wild, SH.; Krone, N.; Doherty, EJ.; Hahner, S.; Han, TS.; Carroll, PV.; Conway, GS.; Rees, PA.; Stimson, RH.; Walker, BR.; Connell, JM.; Ross, RJ. (2010). United Kingdom Congenital Adrenal Hyperplasia Adult Study Executive (CaHASE). Health status of adults with congenital adrenal hyperplasia; a cohort study of 203 patients. *J Clin Endocrinol Metab.* Vol.95, No.11, pp. 5110-5121

Arslanian, SA.; Lewy, V.; Danadian, K.; Saad, R. (2002). Metformin therapy in obese adolescents with polycystic ovary syndrome and impaired glucose tolerance: amelioration of exaggerated adrenal response to adrenocorticotropin with reduction of insulinemia/insulin resistance. *J Clin Endocrinol Metab.* Vol.87, pp. 1555-1559

Bahtiyar, G.; Weiss, K.; Sacerdote, AS. (2007). Novel endocrine disrupter effects of classic and atypical antipsychotic agents and divalproex: induction of adrenal hyperandrogenism reversible with metformin or rosiglitazone. *Endocr Pract* Vol.13, pp. 601-608

Bercovici, JM.; Monguillon, P.; Nahoul, K.; Floch, HH.; Brettes, JP. (1996). Polycystic ovary and Diazoxide. In vivo study. *Ann Endocrinol.* Vol.57, No.4, pp. 235-239

Bilo, L.; Meo, R. (2208). Polycystic ovary syndrome in women using valproate. *Gyneco Endocrinol.* Vol.24, No.10, pp.562-570

Carbunaru, G.; Prasad, P.; Scoccia, B. Shea P, Hopwood N, Ziai F, Chang YT, Myers SE, Mason JI, Pang S. (2004). The hormonal phenotype of non-classic 3-beta-hydroxysteroid dehydrogenase (HSD3B) deficiency in hyperandrogenic females is associated with insulin-resistant polycystic ovary syndrome and is not a variant of inherited HSD3B2 deficiency. *J Clin Endocrinol Metab.* Vol.89, pp. 783-794

Cavalier, E.; Delanaye, P.; Souberbielle, JC.; Radermecker, RP. (2011). Vitamin D and Type 2 diabetes mellitus: Where do we stand? *Diab Metab.* Vol.21, [Epub ahead of print]

Charmandari, E.; Weise, M.; Bornstein, SR.; Eisenhofer, G.; Keil, MF.;, Chrousos, GP.;, Merke, DP. (2002). Children with classical congenital adrenal hyperplasia have elevated serum leptin concentrations and insulin resistance: potential clinical implications. *J Clin Endocrinol Metab.* Vol.87, pp. 2114-2120

Choi, YH.; Cho, SY.; Cho, IR. (2010). The different reduction rates of prostate-specific antigen in dutasteride and finasteride. *Lorean J Urol*, Vol.. 51, No. 10, pp. 704-708.

Connery, LE.; Coursin, DB. (2004). Assessment and therapy of selected endocrine disorders. *Anesthiol Clin North America,* Vol.22, No.1, pp. 93-123

Defronzo, RA.; Triplitt, C.; Qu, Y.; Lewis, MS.; Maggs, D.; Glass, LC. (2010). Effects of exenatide plus rosiglitazone on beta-cell function and insulin sensitivity in subjects with type 2 diabetes on metformin. *Diabetes Care* Vol.33, No.5, pp. 951-957

Derosa, G.; Maffioli, P.; Ferrari, I.; D'Angelo, A.; Fogari, E.; Palumbo, I.; Randazoo, S.; Cicero, AF. (2010). Orlistat and L-carnitine compared to orlistat alone on insulin resistance in obese diabetic patients. *Endoc J,* Vol.57, No.9, pp. 777-786

Dormandy, J.; Bhattacharya, M.; Van Troostenburg de Bruyn, AR. (2009). PROactive investigators. Safety and tolerability of pioglitazone in high-risk patients with type 2 diabetes: an overview of data from PROactive. *Drug Saf,* Vol. 32, No.3, pp. 187-202

Eid, GM.; Cottam, DR.; Velcu, LM.; Mattar, SG.; Korytkowski, MT.; Gosman, G.; Hindi, P.; Schauer, PR. (2005). Effective treatment of polycystic ovarian syndrome with Roux-en-Y gastric bypass. *Surg Obes Relat Dis,* Vol.1, No.2, pp. 77-80

Elkind-Hirsch, K.; Marrioneaux, O.; Bhushan, M.; Vernor, D.; Bhushan, R. (2008). Comparison of single and combined treatment with exenatide and metformin on menstrual cyclicity in overweight women with polycystic ovary syndrome. *J Clin Endocrinol Metab.* Vol.93, No.7, pp. 2670-2678

Feig, DS.; Briggs, GG.; Koren, G. (2007). Oral antidiabetic agents in pregnancy and lactation: a paradigm shift? *Ann Pharmacother.* Vol.41, No.7, pp. 1174-80

Franks, S. (2011). When should an insulin sensitizing agent be used in the treatment of polycystic ovary syndrome? *Clin Endocrinol.* Vol.74, No.2, pp. 148-151

Fujimoto, S.; Kondoh, H.; Yamamoto, Y.; Hisanaga, S.; Tanaka, K. (1990). Holter electrocardiogram monitoring in nephrotic patients during methylprednisolone pulse therapy. *Am J Nephrol,* Vol.10, No.3, pp. 231-236

Gambineri, A.; Patton, L.; De Iasio, R.; Cantelli, B.; Cognini, GE.; Filicori, M.; Barreca, A.; Diamanti- Kandarakis, E.; Pagotto, U.;, Pasquali, R. (2005). Efficacy of octreotide-LAR in dieting women with abdominal and polycystic ovary syndrome. *J Clin Endocrinol Metab.* Vol.90, No.7, pp. 3854-3862

Ghosh, SS.; Massey, HD.; Krieg, R.;Fazelbhoy, ZA.; Ghosh, S.; Sica, DA.; Fakhry, I.; Gehr, TW. (2009). Curcumin ameliorates renal failure in 5/6 nephrectomized rats: role of inflammation. *Am J Physiol Renal Physiol.* Vol.296, No.5, pp. 1146-1157

Glueck, CJ.; Goldenberg, N.; Wang, P.; Loftspring, M.; Sherman, A. (2004). Metformin during pregnancy reduces insulin, insulin resistance, insulin secretion, weight, testosterone and development of gestational diabetes: prospective longitudinal assessment of women with polycystic ovary syndrome from preconception throughout pregnancy. *Hum Reprod,* Vol.19, No.3, pp. 510-521

Gondo, S.; Yanase, T.; Okabe, T.; Tanaka T, Morinaga H, Nomura M, Goto K, Nawata H. (2004). SF-1/Ad4BP transforms primary long-term cultured bone marrow cells into into ACTH-responsive steroidogenic cells *Genes to Cells* Vol.9, No.12, pp. 1239-1247

Hamada, S.; Chin, K.; Hitomi, T.; Oga, T.; Handa, T.; Tuboi, T.; Niimi, A.; Mishima, M. (2011). Impact of nasal continuous positive airway pressure for congenital adrenal hyperplasia with obstructive sleep apnea and bruxism. *Sleep Breath,* Epub 2011 Feb 18 (ahead of print)

Inoue, A.; Sawata, SY.; Taira, K. (2006). Molecular design and delivery of siRNA. *J Drug Target* Vol.14, pp. 448-455

Jakubowicz, DJ.; Iurno, MJ.; Jakubowicz, S.; Roberts, KA.; Nestler, JE. (2002). Effects of metformin on early pregnancy loss in the polycystic ovary syndrome. *J Clin Endocrinol Metab.* Vol.87, No.2, pp. 524-529

Kelly, SN.; McKenna, TJ.; Young, LS. (2004). Modulation of steroidogenic enzymes by orphan nuclear transcriptional regulation may control diverse production of cortisol and androgens in the human adrenal. *J Endocrinol,* Vol.181, pp. 355-3365

Kim, AC.; Hammer, GD. (2007). Adrenocortical cells with stem/progenitor cell properties: recent advances. *Molecular and Cellular Endocrinology,* Epub 2007 Jan 19, pp. 265-266

Kroese, JM.; Mooij, CF.; van der Graaf, M.; Hermus, AR.; Tack, CJ. (2009). Pioglitazone improves insulin resistance and decreases blood pressure in adult patients with congenital adrenal hyperplasia. *Eur J Endocrinol* Vol.161, No.6, pp. 887-894

Ladson, G.; Dodson, WC.; Sweet, SD.; Archibong, AE.; Kunselman, AR.; Demers, LM.; Williams, NI.; Coney, P.; Legro, RS. (2011). The effects of metformin with lifestyle therapy in polycystic ovary syndrome: a randomized double-blind study. *Fertil Steril,* Vol.95, No.3, pp. 1059-1066

Liu, Q.; Adams, L.; Broyde, A.; Fernandez, R.; Baron, AD.; Parkes, DG. (2010). The exenatide analogue AC3174 attenuates hypertension, insulin resistance, and renal dysfunction in Dahl salt-sensitive rats. *Cardiovasc Diabetol* Vol.3, No.9, p. 32

Loechner, KJ.; McLaughlin, JT.; Calikoglu, AS. (2010). Alternative strategies for the treatment of classical congenital adrenal hyperplasia: Pitfalls and promises. *Int J Pediatic Endocrinol,* 2010:670960. Epub 2010 June 24

Lutfallah, C.; Wang, W.; Mason, JI.; Mason, JI.; Chang, YT.; Haider, A.; Rich, B.; Castro-Magana, M.; Copeland, KC.; David, R.; Pang, S. (2002). Newly proposed hormonal criteria via genotypic proof for Type II 3beta-hydroxysteroid dehydrogenase deficiency. *J Clin Endocrinol Metab,* Vol.87, No.6, pp. 2611-2622

Mannelli, M.; Cantini, G.; Poli, G.; Mangoni, M.; Nesi, G.; Canu, L.; Rapizzi, E.; Ercolini, T.; Piccini, V.; Luconi, M. (2010). Role of the PPAR-γ in normal and tumoral pituitary and adrenal cells. *Neuroendocrinology,* Vol.92, pp. 23-27

Mapas-Dimaya, AC.; Agdere, L.; Bahtiyar, G.; Mejía, JO.; Sacerdote, AS. (2008). Metformin-responsive classic salt-losing congenital adrenal hyperplasia due to 21-hydroxylase deficiency: a case report. *Endocr Pract,* Vol.14, pp. 889-891

Merke, DP.; Bornstein, SR. (2005). Congenital adrenal hyperplasia. *Lancet.* Vol.365, No.9477, pp. 2125-2136

Merke, DP. (2008). Approach to the adult with congenital adrenal hyperplasia due to 21-hydroxylase deficiency. *J Clin Endocrinol Metab,* Vol.93, No.3, pp. 653-660

Migrenne, S.; Lacombe, A.; Lefèvre, AL.; Pruniaux, MP.; Guillot, E.; Galzin, AM.; Magnan, C. (2009). Adiponectinis required to mediate rimonabant-induced improvement of insulin sensitivity but not body weight loss in diet-induced obese mice. *Am J Physiol Regul Integr Comp Physiol,* Vol.296, No.4, pp. 929-935

Mooij, CF.; Kroes, JM.; Claahsen-van der Grinten, HL.; Tack, CJ.; Hermus, AR. (2010). Unfavorable trends in cardiovascular and metabolic risk in pediatric and adult patients with congenital adrenal hyperplasia. *Clin Endocrinol,* Vol. 73, No.2, pp. 137-146

Newell-Price, J.; Whiteman, M.; Rostami-Hodjegan, A.; Darzy, K.; Shalet, S.; Tucker, GT.; Ross RJ. (2008). Modified-release hydrocortisone for circadian therapy: a proof-of-principle study in dexamethasone-suppressed normal volunteers. *Clin Endocrinol,* Vol.68, No.1, pp. 130-135

Nissen, SE.; Wolski, K. (2007). Effect of rosiglitazone on the risk of myocardial infarction and death from cardiovascular causes. *N Engl J Med,* Vol.356, No.24, pp. 2457-2471

Nunlee-Bland, G.; Gambhir, K.; Abrams, C.; Abdul, M.; Vahedi, M.; Odonkor, W. (20011). Vitamin D deficiency and insulin resistance in obese African-American adolescents. *J Pediatr Endocrinol Metab,* Vol.24, No.1-2, pp. 29-33

Osehobo, E.; Sacerdote, AS. (1999). Aldosterone Synthase Deficiency; A Newly Described Variant of Non-Classical Congenital Adrenal Hyperplasia. *Program and Abstracts, 81sAnnual Meeting of the Endocrine Society,* June 12-15, 1999, San Diego, CA, p. 586

Osehobo, E.; Shaw, I.; Sacerdote, AS. (2000). Do insulin sensitizers repair the gene defects in non-classical congenital adrenal hyperplasia? *Program and Abstracts of the 82nd Annual Meeting of the Endocrine Society;* June 21-4, 2000; Toronto, Canada. Abstract No. 547

Pall, M.; Azziz, R.; Beires, J.; Pignatelli, D. (2010). The phenotype of hirsute women: a comparison of polycystic ovary syndrome and 21-hydroxylase-deficient nonclassic adrenal hyperplasia. *Ferti Steril,* Vol.94, No.2, pp. 684-689

Panidis, D.; Farmakiotis, D.; Rousso, D.; Koutis, A.; Katsikis, I.; Krassas, G. (2008). Obesity, weight loss, and the polycystic ovary syndrome: effect of treatment with diet and orlistat for 24 weeks on insulin resistance and androgen levels. *Fertil Steril,* Vol.89, No.4, pp. 899-906

Paoletti, AM.; Cagnacci, A.; Depau, GF.; Orrù, M.; Ajossa, S.; Melis, GB. (1996). The chronic administration of cabergoline normalizes androgen secretion and improves menstrual cyclicity in women with polycystic ovary syndrome. *Fertil Steril,* Vol.66, No.4, pp. 527-532

Pijl H, Ohashi S, Matsuda M. (2000). Bromocriptine: a novel approach to the treatment of Type 2 diabetes. *Diab Care,* Vol. 23, pp. 1154-1161

Pittas, AG.; Lau, J.; Hu, FB.; Dawson-Hughes, B. (2007). The role of vitamin D and calcium in type 2 diabetes. A systematic review and meta-analysis. *J Clin Endocrinol Metab,* Vol.92, pp. 2017–2029

Raff, H. (2004). Neonatal dexamethasone therapy: short- and long-term consequences, *Trends Endocrinol Metab,* Vol.15, pp. 351–352

Rashidi, B.; Haghollahi, F.; Shariat, M.; Zaterii, F. (2009). The effects of calcium-vitamin D and metformin on polycystic ovary syndrome: a pilot study. *Taiwan J Obstet Gynecol,* Vol.48, No.2, pp. 142-147

Rieppe, FG.; Sippell, WG. (2007). Recent advances in diagnosis, treatment,, and outcome of congenital adrenal hyperplasia due to 21-hydroxylase deficiency. *Rev Endocr Metab Disord* Vol.8, No. 4, pp. 349-363

Sathyapalan, T.; Cho, LW.; Kilpatrick, ES.; Coady, AM.; Atkin, SL. (2008). A comparison between rimonabant and metformin in reducing biochemical hyperandrogenemia and insulin resistance in patients with polycystic ovary syndrome (PCOS): a randomized open-label parallel study. *Clin Endocrinol,* Vol.69, No.6, pp. 931-935

Sacerdote, AS.; Vergara, R.; Carnegie, B. (1995). Do All Patients with NIDDM Have Late-Onset Congenital Adrenal Hyperplasia? *Program and Abstracts, 76th Annual Meeting of the Endocrine Society:* 350, 1994 (poster presentation).

Sacerdote, AS. Adrenal androgens and NIDDM. *Diabetes Care,* Vol.18, No.2, pp. 278-279

Sacerdote, AS. (2002). Weight-Dependent Expression of Non-Classical Aldosterone Synthase Deficiency. *Program and Abstracts of the 84th Annual Meeting of the Endocrine Society;* June 19-22, 2002, San Francisco, CA, Abstract No. 599

Sacerdote, AS.; Sanchez, JU.; Ogbeide, O.; Slabodkina, L. (2003). Modification of expression of non-classical congenital adrenal hyperplasia by rosiglitazone. *Program and Abstracts of the 85th Annual meeting of the Endocrine Society;* June 19-22, 2003, Philadelphia, PA. Abstract No. 444

Sacerdote, AS. (2004). Modification of expression of non-classical congenital adrenal hyperplasia by pioglitazone. *Program and Abstracts of the 86th Annual Meeting of the Endocrine Society;* June 16-19, 2004; New Orleans, LA. Abstract No. 569

Sacerdote, A.; Girgis, E.; Toossi, A.; Polanco, H.; Bahtiyar, G. (2006). Additional endocrine disrupter effects of highly active anti- retroviral treatment-induction of non-classical adrenal hyperplasia. *Program and Abstracts of the 88th Annual meeting of the Endocrine Society;* June 24-27, 2006, Boston MA. Abstract No. 202

Saygili, F.; Oge, A.; Yilmaz, C. (2005). Hyperinsulinemia ansd insulin insensitivity in women with non-classical congenital adrenal hyperplasia due to 21-hydroxylase deficiency: the relationship between serum leptin levels and chronic hyperinsulinemia. *Hor Res,* Vol.63, No.6, pp. 270-274

Schwartz, SL.; Lai, YL.; Xu, J.; Abby, SL.; Misir, S.; Jones, MR.; Nagendran, S. (2010). The effect of colesevelam hydrochloride on insulin sensitivity and secretion in patients with type 2 diabetes: a pilot study. *Metab Syndr Relat Disord,* Vol.8, No.2, pp. 179-188

Scranton, R.; Cincotta, A. (2010). Bromocriptine—unique formulation of a dopamine agonist for the treatment of type 2 diabetes. *Expert Opin Pharmacother*, Vol.11, No.2, pp. 269-279

Singer, F.; Bhargava, G.; Poretsky, L. (1989). Persistent insulin resistance after normalization of androgen levels in a woman with congenital adrenal hyperplasia. A case report. *J Reprod Med*, Vol.34, No.11, pp. 921-922

Shang, Q.; Saumoy, M.; Holst, JJ.; Salen, G.; Xu, G. (2010). Colesevelam improves insulin resistance in a diet-induced obesity (F-DIO) rat model by increasing the release of GLP-1. *Am J Physiol Gastrointest Liver Physiol*, Vol.298, No.3, pp. G419-424

Speiser, PW.; Serrat, J.; New, MI.; Gertner, JM. (1992). Insulin insensitivity in adrenal hyperplasia due to nonclassical steroid 21-hydroxylase deficiency. *J Clin Endocrinol Metab*, Vol.75, No.6, pp. 1421-1424

Speiser, PW.; Azziz, R.; Baskin, LS.; Ghizzoni, L.; Hensle, TW.; Merke, DP. (2010). Congenital adrenal hyperplasia due to steroid 21-hydroxylase deficiency: an Endocrine Society clinical practice guideline. *J Clin Endocrinol Metab*, Vol.95, No.9. pp. 4133-4160

Spruce, BA.; Kendall-Taylor, P.; Dunlop, W.; Anderson, AJ.; Watson, MJ.; Cook, DB.; Gray, C. (1984). The effect of bromocriptine in the polycystic ovary syndrome. *Clin Endocrinol*, Vol.20, No.4, pp. 481-488

Tai, K.; Need, AG.; Horowitz, M.; Chapman, IM. (2008). Vitamin D, glucose, insulin and insulin sensitivity. *Nutrition*, Vol.24, pp. 279–285

Tasali, E.; Chapoto, F.; Leproult, R.; Whitmore, H.; Ehrmann, DA. (2011). Treatment of obstructive sleep apnea improves cardiometabolic function in young obese women with polycystic ovary syndrome. *J Clin Endocrinol Metab*, Vol. 96, No.2, pp. 365-374

Trapp, CM.; Speiser, PW.; Oberfiled, SE. (2011). Congenital adrenal hyperplasia: an update in children. *Curr Opin Endocrinol Diabetes Obes*, April 13. Epub ahead of print.

Verrotti, A.; D'Egidio, C.; Mohn, A.; Coppola, A.; Parisi, P.; Chiarelli, F. (2011). Antiepileptic drugs, sex hormones, and PCOS. *Epilepsia*, Vol.52, No.2, pp. 199-211

Vgontzas, AN.; Bixler, EO.; Chrousos, GP. (2005). Sleep apnea is a manifestation of the metabolic syndrome. *Sleep Med Rev*, Vol.9, No.3, pp. 211-224

Wehr, E.; Trummer, O.; Giuliani, A.; Gruber, HJ.; Pieber, TR.; Obermayer-Pietsch, B. (2011). Vitamin D-associated polymorphisms are related to insulin resistance and vitamin D deficiency in polycystic ovary syndrome. *Eur J Endocrinol*, Vol.164, No.5, pp. 741-749

White, PC. (1997). Abnormalities of aldosterone synthesis and action in children. *Curr Opin Pediatr*, Vol.9, No.4, pp. 424-430

Yazawa, T.; Mizutani, T.; Yamada, K.; Kawata, H.; Sekiguchi, T.; Yoshino, M.; Kajitani, T.; Shou, Z.; Umezawa, A.; Miyamoto, K. (2006). Differentiation of adult stem cells derived from bone marrow stroma into Leydig or adrenocortical cells. *Endocrinology*, Vol.147, No.9, pp. 4104-4111

Young, MC.; Hughes, IA. (1990). Response to treatment of congenital adrenal hyperplasia in infancy. *Arch Dis Child*, Vol.65, pp. 441-444

Zhang, HJ.; Yang, J.; Zhang, MN.; Liu, CQ.; Xu, M.; Li, XJ.; Yang, SY.; Li, XY. (2010). Metabolic disorders in newly diagnosed young adult female patients with simple virilizing 21-hydroxylase deficiency. *Endocrine* Vol.38, No.2, pp.,260-265

Zimmerman, A.; Grigorescu-Sido, P.; Alkhzouz, C.; Patberg, K.; Bucerzan, S.; Schulze, E.; Zimmerman, T.; Rossmann, H.; Geiss, HC.; Lackner, KJ.; Weber, MM. (2010). Alterations in lipid and carbohydrate metabolism in patients with classical adrenal hyperplasia due to 21- hydroxylase deficiency. *Horm Res Paediatr*, Vol.74, No.1, pp. 41-49

6

From Heavy Menstrual Bleeding to Amenorrhoea and Reversal of Anaemia - Novel, Effective, Intrauterine Levonorgestrel-Releasing Systems for Contraception and Treatment

D. Wildemeersch[1] and A. Andrade[2]
[1]*Outpatient Gynaecological Clinic and IUD Training Center, Ghent*
[2]*Centro de Biologia da Reprodução, Universidade Federal Juiz de Fora, Juiz de Fora*
[1]*Belgium*
[2]*Brazil*

1. Introduction

Menorrhagia, defined as regular but heavy menstrual bleeding of more than 80 ml from a secretory endometrium is a common disorder. The prevalence is between 9% and 28% of women aged 16-45 years and increases with age.[1] Approximately 30% of patients referred for gynaecological treatment are for menorrhagia and half of these women have a hysterectomy within 5 years if conservative treatment (e.g. contraceptive pills, progestogens, fibrinolytic inhibitors and prostaglandin inhibitors) fails. More than one third of these women undergoing hysterectomy have normal uteri.[2,3]

In the USA, more than 600,000 hysterectomies are performed each year of which 30% for excessive menstrual bleeding. In the UK 40% of the 100,000 hysterectomies are performed for that reason. Idiopathic menorrhagia is the most common form of menorraghia when no underlying cause (e.g. uterine and endometrial abnormalities, systemic coagulation defects) can be found. Local defects in the haemostatic mechanism in the endometrium are most probably at the origin of the disorder such as an increased fibrinolytic activity or an imbalance in the different types of prostaglandins.[4]

When menstrual blood loss exceeds 80 ml, the incidence of anaemia (haemoglobin less than 12 g/dl) is increased significantly.[5] Anaemia is one of the most widespread, and most neglected, nutritional deficiency diseases in the world today.[6] Iron deficiency with depletion of iron stores and/or anaemia predisposes the women to ill health and disease. In addition, women with menorrhagia are often prevented from leading normal lives causing severe social embarrassment and repudiation by the partner.

In recent years, new less invasive treatment options have been developed.[7] Endometrial ablation techniques and classical endometrial resection have their value but are costly although significantly cheaper than hysterectomy. They are also irreversible. Second generation endometrial ablation techniques have fewer complications, are quicker and they seem to be more suitable for local anaesthesia than the first generation techniques.

The intrauterine system releasing 20 µg of levonorgestrel (Mirena® LNG-IUS) has shown a dramatic decrease in menstrual blood loss in nearly all women and amenorrhoea in up to 20% or more due to profound endometrial atrophy.[8,9,10]

The present report reviews the reduction of menstrual flow following insertion of the Femilis® LNG-IUS, a new T-shaped hormone-releasing IUS, releasing 20 µg of LNG/day. The report also evaluates other menstrual blood loss (MBL) studies, using the same drug delivery technology for the release of LNG, in which the effect on MBL was assessed with a frameless LNG-IUS, releasing only 14 µg of LNG/day, instead of 20 µg of LNG/day with the framed LNG-IUS. The evaluation is based on 6 clinical studies of which most of them were reported elsewhere.[11,12,13,14,15] The use of the LNG-IUS as first option treatment of menorrhagia or heavy menstrual bleeding is discussed, including for the treatment of iron deficiency anaemia.

2. Materials and methods

2.1 Description of the T-LNG (Femilis®) IUS (Fig. 1) and the frameless FibroPlant®-LNG IUS (Fig. 2)

The T-LNG-IUS (Femilis®, Contrel Drug Delivery Research, Belgium) has a 3-cm long and 2.4-mm wide fibrous delivery system, consisting of a LNG-ethylene vinyl acetate (EVA) core and an EVA rate-controlling membrane that releases approximately 20 µg of LNG daily. The drug compartment is provided with a crossarm fixed to the upper part of the drug delivery rod. The total length of the crossarm is 28 mm. The polyethylene crossarm contains 22% barium sulphate to render it radiopaque. The single tail is made of a 00 gauge polypropylene.

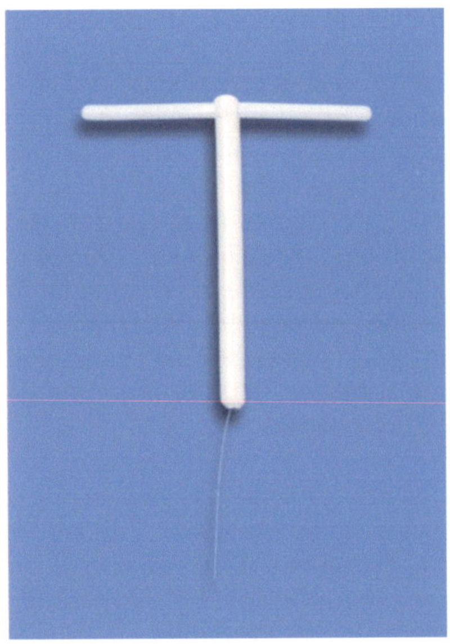

Fig. 1. Femilis®

The FibroPlant® LNG-IUS (Contrel Drug Delivery Research, Belgium) consists of a fibrous delivery system of 3-cm long and 1.2 mm in diameter that releases 14 µg of LNG daily. The fibrous delivery system is fixed to an anchoring filament by means of a metal clip positioned 1 cm from the anchoring knot. The anchoring knot at the proximal end of the thread is implanted into the myometrium of the uterine fundus using an insertion instrument, thus permanently securing the implant in the uterine cavity.

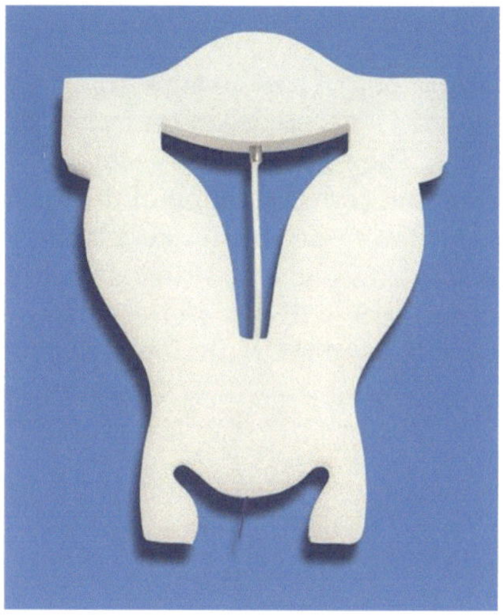

Fig. 2. FibroPlant®

In vitro studies show that the rate of LNG-release is constant over several years (zero-order), except for the first two months of use, and is similar to the in vitro release rate of the Mirena® LNG-IUS. The duration of release is at least five years with the Femilis® LNG-IUS and at least three years with the FibroPlant® LNG-IUS. The in vitro release studies and other pharmacological analyses were conducted in collaboration with the Polymer Research Group, Department of Chemistry, University of Ghent, Ghent, Belgium and with the Analytical Pharmaceutical Chemistry of the Department of Pharmacy, University of Liège, Belgium.

2.2 Insertion technique (Fig. 3 and Fig. 4)

Femilis®

The T-LNG-IUS (Femilis®) is inserted using the 'push-in' technique. Notably, upon entering the uterine cavity the crossarm unfolds immediately, thus minimising the risk of perforation.

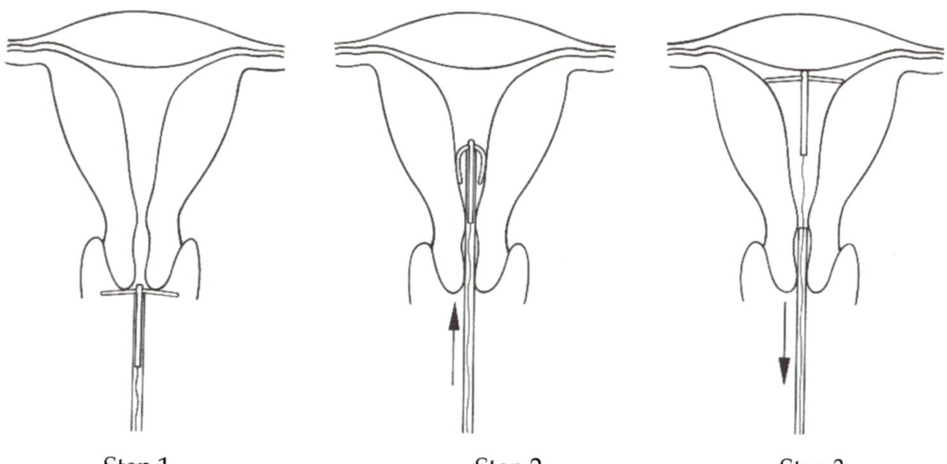

Fig. 3. Insertion procedure of Femilis®.

FibroPlant®

The anchoring knot at the proximal end of the thread is implanted into the myometrium of the uterine fundus using the standard GyneFix® insertion technique, thus permanently securing the implant in the uterine cavity. The stainless steel metal clip allows ultrasound and X-ray visibility of the system thus enabling correct location of the system in the uterine cavity, both at insertion and at follow-up. The fibrous delivery system is also visible on ultrasound.

When compared with "framed" drug delivery systems such as the Mirena® and Femilis® LNG-IUS, the FibroPlant® LNG-IUS will be seen to have no frame. It is, therefore, completely flexible, with the ability to adapt to uterine cavities of every size and shape.

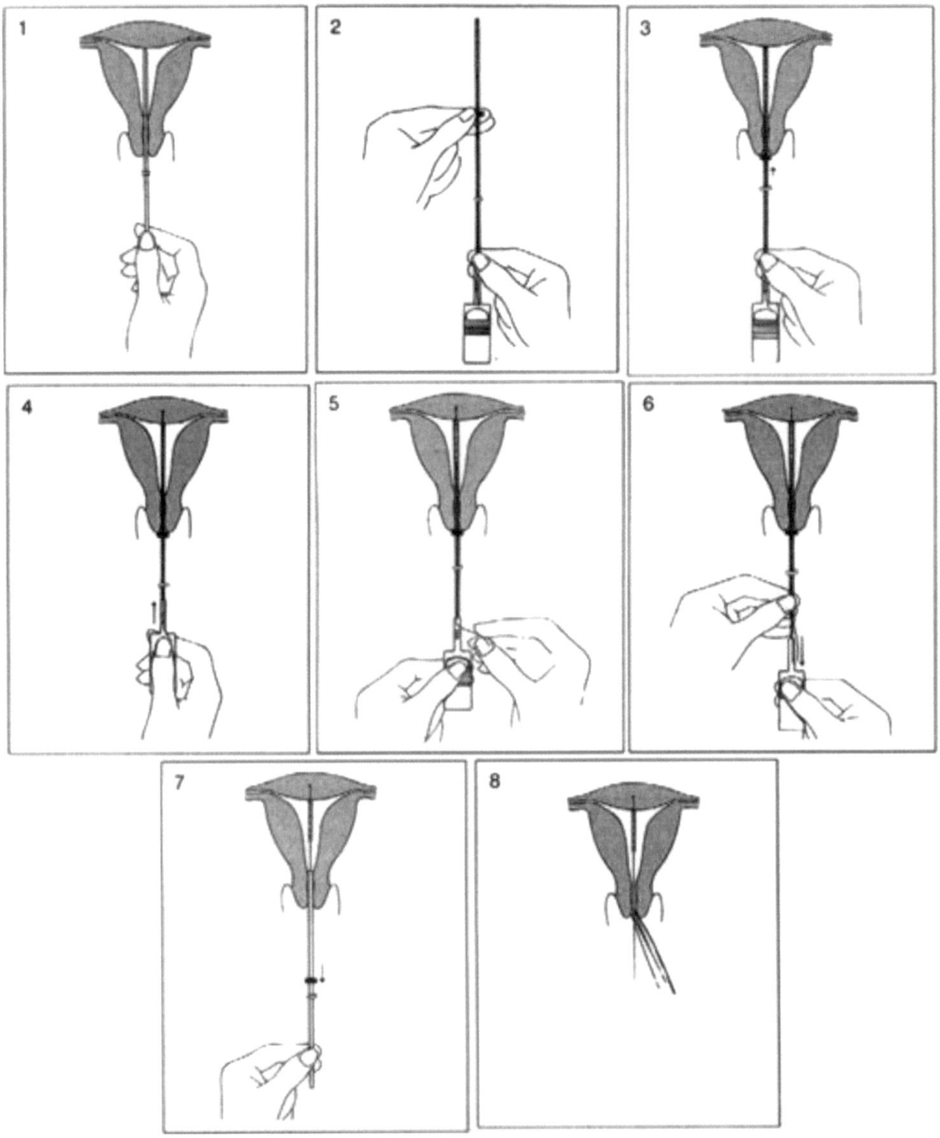

Fig. 4. Insertion procedure of FibroPlant® is identical with the insertion procedure of the frameless GyneFix® copper-releasing IUD (See video insertion on www.wildemeersch.com).

2.3 Study population and menstrual blood loss assessment techniques

Study 1: Femilis® in women with and without idiopathic menorrhagia (assessed by the visual menstrual score technique): Women less than 48 years of age at study enrollment with normal and with heavy menstrual periods were admitted into the study. Women with significant fibromyomas (>3 cm), or other uterine pathology, were excluded form the study. Women were followed-up for at least 12 months.

A visual assessment technique was used as described by Janssen.[3] Information on menstrual bleeding was obtained by interview retrospectively using a pictorial chart to describe the degree to which the sanitary wear was soiled. A score was calculated by multiplying the number of slightly, moderately and heavily soiled pads and tampons by one, five and 20 for pads and one, 5 and 10 for tampons, respectively, according to their degree of staining (Fig. 5). The visual assessment technique does not yield an exact flow in ml, but, in practice, the sensitivity and specificity is reasonably high and superior to a women's subjective assessment of MBL. For purposes of evaluating the effect of treatment, the visual assessment technique is highly practical compared with the quantitative method, described below, as women no longer have to submit sanitary wear to the laboratory.

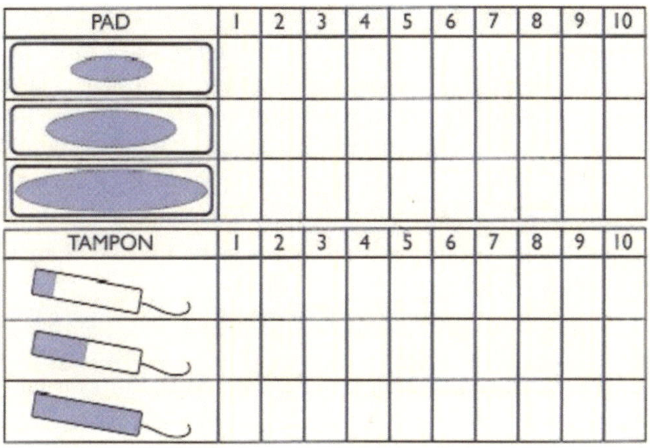

Fig. 5. Pictorial chart for the evaluation of menstrual blood loss.

Study 2: Femilis® in women with and without heavy menstrual bleeding (HMB) (assessed by the quantitative alkaline haematin technique): 14 Brazilian women participated in this menstrual blood loss study (ongoing study). In this study, 6 months results are available in 13 of them. MBL was quantified according to the technique first described by Hallberg and Nilsson[16], adapted by Shaw[17] and modified by Newton[18] before insertion (baseline controls) of the IUS and after 3, and 6 months. Women were instructed to carefully collect their menstrual tampons and bring them to the laboratory in opaque plastic bags as soon as bleeding ended, as described previously.[19] Serum ferritin was also measured at the same intervals as above.

Study 3: FibroPlant® LNG-IUS in women with normal and heavy menstruation (assessed by the quantitative alkaline haematin technique): Menstrual blood loss studies were conducted in 40 Brazilian FibroPlant® LNG users with normal and heavy menstrual bleeding. Women were followed-up for at 3, 6, 12 and 24 months. MBL was quantified according to the technique described above. Serum ferritin was also measured at the same intervals as above.

Study 4: FibroPlant® LNG-IUS in women with idiopathic menorrhagia (visual menstrual score technique): The efficacy of the FibroPlant® LNG-IUS in reducing menstrual blood loss was tested in 12 Belgian women between 17 and 43 years of age suffering from idiopathic menorrhagia using the visual bleeding score (score >185) as described above. Women were followed-up for one year.

Study 5: FibroPlant® LNG-IUS in women with idiopathic menorrhagia (visual menstrual score technique): Thirty-two insertions were performed in fertile women between 31 and 51 years of age for the treatment of menorrhagia as well as for contraceptive purposes. Fifteen women were fitted with the FibroPlant® LNG-IUS immediately following removal of a copper-bearing IUD, the GyneFix® IUD, who developed excessive bleeding. To discriminate between menorrhagia and normal menstrual blood loss, women were evaluated using the visual assessment technique. The trial covers a period from a minimum of 1 month up to 23 months.

Study 6: FibroPlant® LNG-IUS in women with menorrhagia associated with intrauterine fibroids (visual menstrual score technique): Fourteen insertions were performed in premenopausal women between 39 and 48 years of age for the treatment of menorrhagia in the presence of uterine fibroids. The effect on menstrual blood loss was evaluated using the visual assessment technique. Women were followed-up for at least 12 months.

The use of the LNG-releasing IUS was approved by the Ethics Committee of the University of Ghent, Belgium and written informed consent was obtained. The quantitative MBL studies were approved by the Ethics Committee of the University of Juiz de Fora, Brazil. Prior to the insertion procedure, a medical history was taken and pelvic examination was carried out and the patient was checked for any clinical signs of sexually transmitted diseases. A transvaginal ultrasound examination was conducted to check for uterine pathology. In the fibroid MBL study (Study 6), the uterine fibroids were classified clinically and ultrasonographically as follows:

Type I: single or multiple small intramural and subserosal fibroids (<3 cm). No evidence of submucosal fibroids.

Type II: single or multiple intramural and subserosal fibroids (3-6 cm). No evidence of submucosal fibroids.

Type III: single or multiple intramural and subserosal fibroids (>6 cm). No evidence of submucosal fibroids.

Type IV: single or multiple intramural and subserosal fibroids. Suspicion or evidence of submucosal fibroids.

Following insertion, a transvaginal ultrasound (TVU) was performed to locate the device in the uterus. An admission form was completed.

2.4 Follow-up

Women were followed-up at 1, (3), 6, and 12 months following insertion of the LNG-IUS and six-monthly or yearly thereafter. They were asked about their bleeding patterns and about side effects or adverse reactions. A gynaecological examination was performed as well as a transvaginal ultrasound to locate the device. A follow-up form was completed.

2.5 Data collection, monitoring and analysis

Data were recorded on standard pre-coded forms at admission, at each scheduled and unscheduled follow-up visit, and upon discontinuation from the study. All data were sent to

the data-coordinating centre at the Department of Medical Informatics and Statistics, University Hospital, Ghent, Belgium, for statistical data analysis, except the quantitative menstrual blood loss studies which was analysed at the Department of Statistics, Centro de Biologia da Reprodução, Universidade Federal Juiz de Fora, Brazil.
The statistical significance in the studies using the visual assessment technique was calculated according to the *Wilcoxon's Signed Rank test*, $p<0.05$ denoting significance.
In the quantitative MBL study, all comparisons were made by means of the *Chi-square test or the Student's t-test*, $p<0.05$ indicating significance. The coefficient of correlation was used to determine the strength of the relationship between the pairs of variables.
The statistical significance in the studies using the visual assessment technique was calculated according to the *Wilcoxon's Signed Ranks test*, $p<0.05$ denoting significance.

3. Results

Study 1: Femilis® LNG-IUS in women with and without idiopathic menorrhagia assessed by the visual menstrual score technique: The trial covers a period from a minimum of four months to more than 30 months of IUS use. MBL scores dropped significantly during the observation period in all women except one. The median menstrual score at baseline in women with normal menstrual bleeding (score <185) was 140 (range 80-160) and dropped to a median score of five (range 0-150) at the last follow-up, a decrease of 96%. In women with hemorrhagic bleeding (score ≥185) at baseline, menstrual flow dropped from a median score of 232 (range 185-450) at baseline to a median score of three (range 0-50) at the last follow-up visit, a decrease of 99%. Twenty women developed amenorrhoea (33%), 10 in the group of women with normal menstruation and 10 in those women with menorrhagia. Most of the remaining women had strong oligomenorrhea requiring the use of a few panty-liners only. In one woman, MBL did not decrease for any apparent reason, thus requiring further evaluation (Table 1).

	Total (n=60)		Normal menses (n=28)		Menorrhagia (n=32)	
	MS at insertion	MS at last follow-up	MS at insertion	MS at last follow-up	MS at insertion	MS at last follow-up
Median	200	5	140	5	232	3
SD	87.5	21.5	25.7	29.8	75.7	9.4
Minimum	80	0	80	0	185	0
Maximum	450	150	160	150	450	50

Wilcoxon matched-pairs signed-rank test: $p<0.001$ (highly significant).

Table 1. Visual menstrual bleeding scores (MS) before and during treatment (observation from 4 months to 31 months) in 60 Femilis users (all women)

Study 2: Femilis® in women with and without heavy menstrual bleeding (HMB) assessed by the quantitative alkaline haematin technique)(ongoing study): Menstrual blood loss reduced from a mean baseline menstrual volume of 47.6 ml to a mean volume of 1.1 ml after 6 months. Ferritin values increased from a mean value of 74.6 ng/ml at baseline controls to a mean level of 93.5 ng/ml after 6 months of use. Amenorrhoea occurred in all women after 6 months of use, except in one woman (Table 2).

	MBL mean (N)	FERRITIN mean (N)
Baseline controls	47.6 (14)	74.6 (14)
Interval 6 months	1.1 (13)	93.5 (13)

MBL - in ml Ferritin - in ng/ml
Amenorrhoea: all women, except one.

Table 2. Menstrual blood loss quantification (ml) and serum ferritin levels (ng/ml) in 14 Femilis-LNG users compared with controls (preliminary results; study ongoing)

Study 3: FibroPlant® LNG-IUS in women with normal and excessive menstruation assessed by the quantitative alkaline haematin technique: Quantitative menstrual blood loss studies were conducted in 40 Brazilian FibroPlant® users with normal and heavy menstrual bleeding. Menstrual blood loss reduced from a mean baseline menstrual volume of 29.7 ± 2.2 ml to a mean volume of 1.5 ± 2.8 ml after 24 months. Ferritin values increased from a mean baseline value of 31.1 ± 3.2 ng/ml at baseline controls of the LNG-IUS to a mean level of 72.5 ± 2.1 ng/ml after 24 months of use. Differences in menstrual volume and ferritin levels are highly significant ($p<0.0005$) (Table 3). Amenorrhoea occurred in 80% of women out of 40 after 24 months of use.

	MBL mean ± SD (N)	HGB mean ± SD (N)	FERRITIN mean ± SD (N)
Baseline controls	29.7 ± 2.2 (40)	12.4 ± 0.9 (40)	31.1 ± 3.2 (40)
Interval 3 months	3.3 ± 3.6 (39)*	12.5 ± 0.9 (39)	37.1 ± 2.8 (39)*
Interval 6 months	2.0 ± 3.1 (40)*	12.5 ± 0.9 (40)	47.8 ± 2.2 (40)*
Interval 12 months	1.7 ± 2.5 (39) *	12.4 ± 0.8 (40)	56.2 ± 2.1 (40) *
Interval 24 months	1.5 + 2.8 (40)*	12.7 + 1.1 (40)	72.5 ± 2.1 (40)*

MBL in ml HGB - Ferritin in ng/ml
* $p<0.0005$ Observation: due to skewed distribution MBL and Ferritin values were log transformed before calculations
Amenorrhoea (months): 3: 18 users = 45%; 6: 27 users = 67.5%; 12: 28 users = 70%; 24: 32 users = 80%
MBL: pre-insertion: mean 29.7 ± 2.2ml (variation: 3.6 – 90.0 ml)
At 24 months: mean 1.5 ± 2.8ml (variation: 0 – 29.7ml)

Table 3. Menstrual blood loss quantification (ml) and serum ferritin levels (ng/ml) in 40 FibroPlant-LNG users compared with controls

Study 4: FibroPlant® LNG-IUS in women with idiopathic menorrhagia assessed by the visual menstrual score technique: The results are presented in Table 4. All women reported a marked reduction in menstrual blood loss which started from the first menstrual period following insertion of the IUS. Bleeding reduced further over the next months until the 6th month. No amenorrhoea occurred. The difference in menstrual bleeding was highly significant ($p=0.002$) which resulted in a significant increase in ferritin levels ($p=0.002$).

	Before insertion	at 12 months
Median MS ± SD	325.0 ± 122.2	12.5 ± 42.8*
Mean ferritin level ± SD	19.8 ±10.1	44.5 ± 22.2*

Wilcoxon matched-pairs signed-ranks test: *p=0.002 (highly significant)

Table 4. Visual menstrual bleeding scores (MS) and ferritin levels (ng/l) before and during treatment (observation period 12 months) in 12 FibroPlant® users with menorrhagia (score >185).

Study 5: FibroPlant® LNG-IUS in women with idiopathic menorrhagia assessed by the visual menstrual score technique: All women reported greatly reduced bleeding (Table 5). The mean bleeding score before treatment was 338 (185-740) in the group with no prior IUD use and 368 (185-890) in the group with prior IUD use, respectively, and dropped to a mean score of 70 (range 5-210) in the 'no prior IUD use' group and to a mean score of 52 (3-150) in the 'prior IUD use' group, respectively after 1 to 23 months follow-up which is highly statistically significant ($p<0.001$). There was no statistical difference in bleeding scores before and during treatment between the two groups of women with or without prior copper IUD use.

A. Before treatment

	No prior IUD use	Prior IUD use
n	17	15
Mean	337.9	368.0
St. Dev.	139.2	172.0
Median	324.2	328.8
Minimum	185	185
Maximum	740	890

Mann-Whitney U-test: p=0.63 (NS)

B. During treatment

	No prior IUD use	Prior IUD use
n	17	15
Mean	70.0	52.3
St. Dev.	52.8	51.3
Median	62.5	41.3
Minimum	5	3
Maximum	210	150

Mann-Whitney U-test: p=0.31 (NS)

Table 5. Analysis of the Visual Bleeding Scores comparison between the group with prior IUD use (n = 15) and the group with no prior IUD use (n = 17). A. Before treatment. B: During treatment

Study 6: Femilis® LNG-IUS in women with menorrhagia associated with intrauterine fibroids assessed by the visual menstrual score technique: All women reported greatly reduced bleeding, except one. In two women, the treatment failed although both reported reduced bleeding. One failure was due to the presence of a large endometrial polyp. This patient underwent hysterectomy. The other women had submucosal fibroids. She refused hysterectomy and is continuing treatment. In the other 12 patients, reduction of bleeding was apparent after one month of treatment and tended to decrease further over the next months to stabilize afterwards. The mean bleeding score before treatment was 465 (185-960) and dropped to a mean score of 100 (range 5-300) after treatment which is highly statistically significant ($p<0.001$) (Table 6). In 8 women, the bleeding reduced to very low scores.

	Age	VBS before treatment	VBS during treatment
Mean	45	455	100
Std Deviation	3	210	85
Median	45	410	71
Range	39 - 49	185 - 960	5 - 300

Table 6. Descriptive statistics: age and visual bleeding scores (VBS) before and during treatment

4. Discussion and conclusion

The intrauterine release of LNG alters the function of the endometrium. This phenomenon offers special benefits for users and a manner of local intrauterine therapy.

The reduction of menstrual blood loss is based on the antiproliferative action of the LNG-IUS on the endometrium. The morphology of the endometrium is considerably altered, showing massive decidualization of the stroma, atrophic glands, and sometimes atrophy of the whole functional layer.[20] Normal endometrium during the menstrual cycle produces many highly active compounds (e.g., prostaglandins, estrogen, and estro-progestogen-induced growth factors and other bioactive peptides). In the endometrium suppressed by LNG, the production of these compounds is down regulated. On the other hand, progestogen stimulates the synthesis of other factors such as prolactine receptor, cyclooxygenase-2, and insulin-like growth factor-binding protein-1.[21,22] Furthermore, a significant increase in uterine artery resistance occurs in LNG-IUS users 1 year after insertion which might contribute in reducing menstrual blood flow with the LNG-IUS.[23]

4.1 Treatment of idiopathic menorrhagia

The Mirena® LNG-IUS, releasing 20 µg of LNG/day has been compared with other medication in the treatment of menorrhagia.[24,25,26] Overall, the Mirena® LNG-IUS has been found to be more effective than conventional medication and treatment is also more economic. It was also found that the LNG-IUS was much more effective in reducing the mean MBL below the upper limit of normal MBL (<80 ml). When compared with transcervical endometrial resection (TCRE), both methods are equally effective. However,

endometrial destruction is not always complete. It could, therefore be beneficial to use the hormonal IUS in combination with endometrial destruction. The LNG-IUS, inserted just after the procedure, can be used to improve the results of endometrial resection. Maia et al.[27] reported the results of an interesting study. They investigated 106 women with HMB. After endometrial resection, the women were randomized into two groups, 53 women in each. Women in the treatment group were fitted with Mirena®. In this group, amenorrhoea was achieved in 72% of cases after 3 months, in 89% after 6 months and in 100% after 1 year. In the resection-only group, the corresponding numbers were 19%, 17% and 9%, and in this group, 19% of the women underwent a second resection.
Endometrial resection requires a specialist with endoscopic skills, and to be safe, well-equipped operation facilities. Endometrial ablation is associated with a higher risk of perioperative and long-term complications than use of a LNG-IUS. The cost over 5 years is high because of recurrences and hysterectomies. These are not problems in connection with the LNG-IUS. However, the most important difference between operative therapy and use of the LNG-IUS is that fertility is lost after the former treatment. On the other hand, women at risk for pregnancy and undergoing endometrial ablation should use effective contraception or consider being surgically sterilized, whereas the LNG-IUS provides effective contraception, and treats heavy menstrual bleeding.
In comparison with hysterectomy, morbidity (readmission for serious adverse events) is much higher in women undergoing surgery. In a recently conducted nationwide study in the UK, it was found that hysterectomy for benign indications, irrespective of surgical technique, increases the risk for subsequent stress-urinary-incontinence surgery.[28] In addition, the overall costs of surgery are about three times higher in women undergoing hysterectomy than in women using the Mirena® LNG-IUS.[29]
A recent Cochrane review on surgical versus medical therapy for heavy menstrual bleeding concluded that the Mirena® LNG-IUS provides a better alternative to surgery than oral medication.[30] Although hysterectomy is a definite treatment for heavy menstrual bleeding, it does not improve the overall quality of life significantly more than the LNG-IUS and can cause serious complications. Questions remains, however, about the long term clinical effectiveness of all the treatments; evidence from trials with longer term follow-up (four years or more) is limited. The LNG-IUS, in particular, versus alternative forms of surgical treatment requires further research.
The MBL studies reviewed in this report conducted with the T-shaped (Mirena®-like) LNG IUS, Femilis®, releasing 20 µg of LNG/day, and with the "frameless" FibroPlant® LNG- IUS, releasing 14 µg of LNG/day, in women with a normal menstrual pattern and in women with idiopathic menorrhagia, found a similar drastic reduction in MBL as in the studies conducted with the Mirena® LNG-IUS. Some of these studies are conducted over more than 5 years without recurrence of episodes of heavy periods.

4.2 Abnormal uterine bleeding in women certain subgroups of women

4.2.1 Abnormal uterine bleeding in women with hemostatic disorders or using anticoagulant therapy

The most common underlying bleeding disorder is von Willebrand's disease, which occurs in only 1% to 2% of the general population but in approximately 13% of women with excessive menstrual bleeding. The diagnosis of von Willebrand's disease in healthy females with excessive menses is a true challenge to the gynaecological community. In such women, bleeding disorders might be "mild," with menorrhagia being the only apparent clinical impact of the disorder. The diagnosis of von Willebrand's disease and other bleeding disorders might have an important impact on a woman and her family. It should be emphasized that gynaecologists should consider causes of excessive menstruation that are "outside the uterus" and that some pathology, such as subserosal or intramural leiomyomas, might indeed be asymptomatic. For women who are diagnosed with von Willebrand's disease and heavy menstrual bleeding, there is likely a benefit from the provision of the LNG-IUS.[31,32] Thus, the LNG-IUS appears to be an effective long-term treatment for HMB in women with inherited bleeding disorders (IBDs) in general. Also women having anticoagulant therapy could benefit from the LNG-IUS.[33,34]

4.2.2 Excessive menstrual bleeding in adolescents

Menstrual disorders are common in adolescent girls in general. It commonly begins at menarche and can present acutely. This is usually secondary to anovulatory cycles caused by the immaturity of the hypothalamic-pituitary-ovarian axis. The condition adversely affects the QOL of affected adolescents. It can cause significant distress and discomfort in adolescent girls. It also has major health implications, such as iron deficiency anaemia and the need for hospitalization and blood transfusion in severe cases. It can affect their school attendance and performance. Treatment options include tranexamic acid, the combined oral contraceptive pill, the LNG-IUS, and specific hemostatic therapies, such as desmopressin and clotting factor replacement, if associated with inherent bleeding disorders.[35] These conservative treatment options should seek to avoid surgical intervention. When the LNG-IUS is selected, care should be taken to insert a device that fits in the usually small uterine cavity of these young women to maximize acceptance and continuation of use.

4.3 Heavy bleeding in intrauterine device users

Copper-releasing intrauterine devices may induce longer, heavier, and more painful periods. Pain and heavy menstrual bleeding are common reasons for discontinuing use of an intrauterine device within the first year. A recent Cochrane review evaluated data from 15 randomised controlled trials investigating the effect of NSAIDs on treatment or prevention of pain and bleeding due to an intrauterine contraceptive device.[36] Data from prevention trials were inconsistent. In otherwise asymptomatic women NSAIDs reduced pain or bleeding (or both) in three studies, did not differ from placebo in two studies, and reduced bleeding but not pain in another. A large trial of 2019 first time users in Chile did not support the prophylactic use of ibuprofen compared with placebo to reduce rates of removal of devices because of pain or bleeding.[37] Pain and/or abnormal, erratic or heavy menstrual bleeding is often caused by disharmony between the IUD and the uterine cavity (Figure 6). Recent 3-D sonography studies compared women with abnormally and those with normally located IUDs with respect to their indication for sonography and found that the proportion of patients whose principal indication for sonography was bleeding, pain or bleeding and pain were significantly greater in those with an abnormally located IUD, including imbedded IUDs, compared with those whose IUD was not located abnormally on 3-D sonography.[38,39] Clinical trials demonstrated, for the first time, the absence of a significant effect of the tiny GyneFix® IUD on menstrual blood loss due to its very small size and optimal harmony with the uterine cavity, leaving the cavity totally undisturbed.[40] This is important since abnormal bleeding and pain are the two major reasons for IUD discontinuation.[41] In a Swedish study in CuT380A IUD users an increase in MBL was shown which ranged between 50 and 60%.[42]

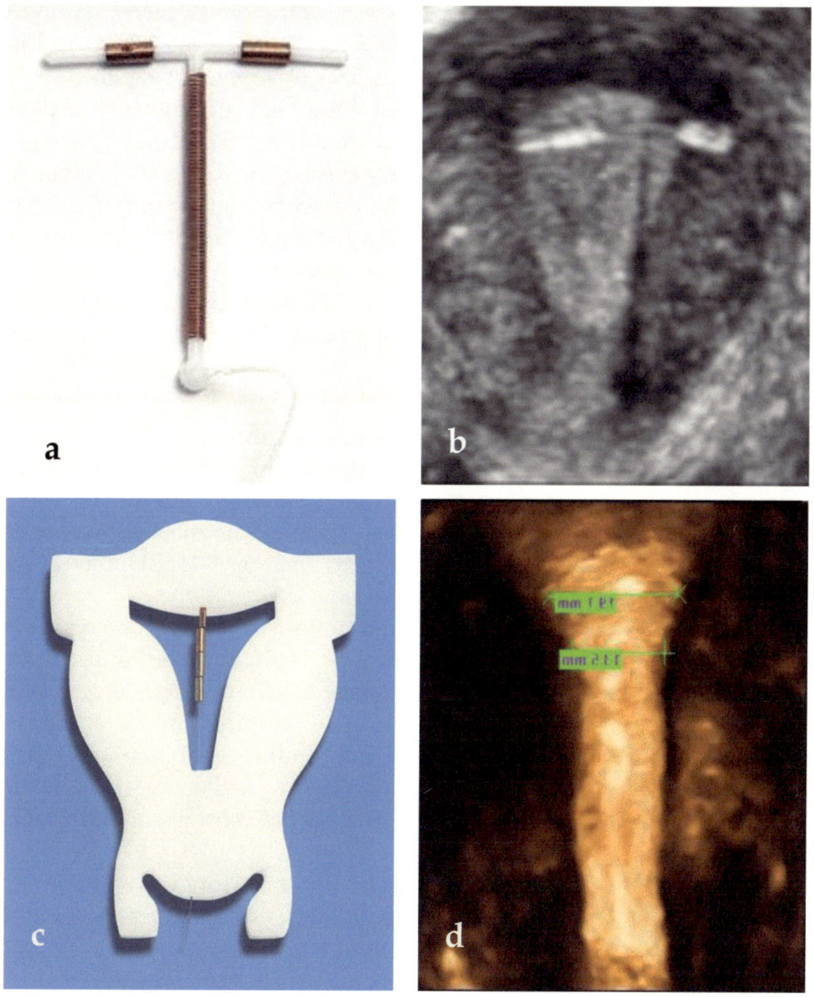

Fig. 6. a) Paragard® IUD; b) 3-D sonography of Paragard® in small uterine cavity of which the left arm penetrates the uterine wall (courtesy of Dr. B. Benacerraf); frameless GyneFix® IUD in foam uterus; 3-D sonographic picture of GyneFix® in narrow uterine cavity (courtesy of Dr. S. Jandi).

Many women can tolerate alterations in bleeding with copper-releasing IUDs. However, if the menstrual bleeding disturbances are causing discomfort or are too heavy, removal of the IUD will be requested. Of great importance are the long-term implications of excessive menstrual blood loss on iron stores with progressive development of iron depletion in IUD users, especially in developing country regions where the recipients of this contraceptive method are commonly of high parity and poor nutritional status. Kivijarvi et al. found clinical anaemia in 10% of users of copper IUDs after 12 months exposure and iron deficiency, as judged by the ferritin levels, could be demonstrated in 20%.[43] The effect of

MBL on iron stores was studied in Sweden which showed that the prevalence of iron deficiency anaemia doubled when MBL was between 60 and 80 ml and tripled when MBL was greater than 80 ml.[43,44] A significant drop in haemoglobin levels already occurs in women with an average menstrual blood loss of 66 ml over 12 menstrual cycles of IUD use.[45] The vulnerability of women in certain less developing parts of the world is indicated by the presence of iron deficiency in as many as 50% of women using an IUD, if a dietary supplement is not provided. It is probable that about 10% of women using an IUD risk secondary anaemia, especially those who bleed more than 80 ml per period. It has been suggested that an increased risk of iron deficiency exists even with a 40 ml blood loss.[46]

The main challenge of intrauterine contraceptive developers is to minimize menstrual side effects of IUDs without affecting efficacy and to reduce menstrual blood loss to enhance the health benefits of the method. Especially for women with low body iron stores, there is an order of preference for IUD use to minimize menstrual blood loss. The choice should first be a progestogen-releasing IUS, then a copper IUD which has the least effect on menstrual bleeding.

4.4 Treatment of menorrhagia associated with uterine fibroids

Although the main therapeutic approach in women with uterine leiomyomata remains surgery, several conservative medical treatments have been tested. The role of GnRH agonists in the treatment of uterine leiomyomas is limited as most leiomyomas return to their initial size within 4 months of cessation of the therapy.[47] GnRH agonists are mainly useful when used preoperatively to reduce the myoma size.

Treatment of leiomyomas with progestogens and antiestrogens is based on the suggestion that leiomyomas are ovarian steroid dependent. The result, however, of progesterone have been poor and no studies have ever demonstrated the benefit of progesterone alone.[48]

Tamoxifen inhibits breast cancer cells by its great affinity for the estrogen receptor. However, on the endometrial level tamoxifen may induce endometrial hyperplasia and endometrial cancer. While acting as an anti-oestrogen on the breast, tamoxifen has an opposite effect on the endometrium as it acts as a partial estrogen agonist, rather than as an antagonist.[49]

To avoid systemic systems, local therapy might optimize innovative approaches. Local therapy has been widely used for contraception but it has not been used to control leiomyoma symptoms. Intrauterine treatment might target myoma specific symptoms better and be more effective in reducing pelvic pressure due to the size of the tumor, and abnormal uterine bleeding. The success rate is less consistent especially in the presence of submucosal fibroids. The reduction in MBL in women with uterine fibroids was also confirmed in two recently published studies using the Mirena® LNG-IUS.[50,51] The results are similar with those reported by Wildemeersch et al.[12] Haemoglobin and ferritin levels increased significantly over 1 year of use. It appears that in women with a normal uterine cavity, a success rate in terms of a significant reduction in MBL close to 100% can be guaranteed.

The study conducted in women with significant fibroids (Study 6) confirms the previous results in women with menorrhagia with normal uteri. Twelve out of 14 women admitted in the study were successfully treated. The treatment, however, was unsuccessful in two women due to abnormalities present in the uterine cavity. It follows that, if reduction of bleeding cannot be obtained, the presence of intracavitary pathology (e.g. submucous fibroids, polyps) should be suspected. Treatment failure in the presence of submucosal fibroids is caused by blood vessels which proliferate in the endometrium overlying the fibroid which can cause 'heavy' bleeding. These vessels are not present in subserosal fibroids. This study does not suggest that LNG-release in the uterine cavity is capable of reducing the size of the myomas in women at reproductive age. The LNG-IUS significantly reduces uterine volume in women with menorrhagia with and without leiomyoma. The absence of significant reduction in the volume of leiomyomas was confirmed by others.[52] Decrease in size of leiomyomas is usually seen in menopausal women. In a study conducted by Inki and colleagues, no marked change was noted in the mean size of the fibroids. Further evaluation revealed that some had grown and some had shrunk.[53] Maruo and colleagues suggested that progesterone may have dual actions on uterine leiomyoma growth. By up regulating some endometrial proteins and down regulating tumor necrosis factor α, progesterone can stimulate leiomyoma growth, and by down regulating insulin-like growth factor-1 expression, inhibit growth.[54] Local autocrine or paracrine growth factor balance around each fibroid may define the direction of the effect.

Local delivery of other drugs such as mifepristone or another progesterone receptor modulator (PRM), with strong antiprogestogen activity and antiestrogenic effect at the endometrial level, may be more suitable to reduce the size of the fibroid tumors.

An additional advantage of the LNG-IUS is the highly appeasing effect of the treatment in women with dysmenorrhoea. Wildemeersch and colleagues showed a highly beneficial effect in women with dysmenorrhoea, confirming other studies, conducted with the frameless LNG-IUS in women with primary and secondary dysmenorrhoea.[55]

4.5 Treatment of anaemia due to heavy menstrual bleeding

Excessive MBL (>80 ml) is the most common cause of iron deficiency anaemia in women.[56] Many women, especially in developing countries, start their reproductive years with inadequate iron stores. Because of the closely spaced pregnancies, they have little time to build up their haemoglobin levels.[4] Each pregnancy makes them more vulnerable to serious ill health and death. A survey conducted by the World Health Organization reported a 19% prevalence rate of menorrhagia in 14 developing countries.[57]

An immediate and cost-effective solution is to provide women with a progestogen-releasing device to minimize MBL, especially for women with low body iron stores which will result in improved haemoglobin and ferritin levels. The use of the LNG-IUS is, therefore, an economical and logical approach when compared with alternatives such as hysterectomy or endometrial ablation.[6,25,58] The simultaneous provision of a long-acting and effective contraceptive may also be of substantial benefit to women.

5. Conclusion

We conclude with NICE (National Institute Clinical Excellence)[59]:

Drug treatment

"If history and investigations indicate that pharmaceutical treatment is appropriate and either hormonal or nonhormonal treatments are acceptable, treatments should be considered in the following order:

- Levonorgestrel-releasing intrauterine system, provided long-term (at least 12 months) use is anticipated.
- Tranexamic acid or non-steroidal anti-inflammatory drugs (NSAIDs) or combined oral contraceptives (COCs).

- Norethisterone (15 mg) daily from days 5 to 26 of the menstrual cycle, or injected long-acting progestogens."

"If hormonal treatments are not acceptable to the woman, then either tranexamic acid or NSAIDs can be used."

Surgery

"In women with heavy menstrual bleeding alone, with uterus no bigger than a 10-week pregnancy, endometrial ablation should be considered preferable to hysterectomy." The report makes clear that hysterectomy should only be considered as a last option. Commenting at its launch, Mary Ann Lumsden, a consultant in gynecology and chairwoman of the NICE guidelines development group that produced the report, said: "In the early 1990s it was estimated that at least 60 percent of women presenting with heavy menstrual bleeding would have a hysterectomy to treat the problem, often as a first-line treatment and without discussion of any alternative options. This should now be rare as it is fundamental that all women with heavy periods know there is a range of treatment options, many of which don't require surgery."

An additional advantage of the LNG-IUS is that it may also be beneficial in women with endometriosis, adenomyosis, fibroids and endometrial hyperplasia, conditions which are frequently associated with menorrhagia.[60,61,62]

Most patients are likely to select a non-invasive treatment. Avoiding major surgery, combined with no hospitalization and quick recovery, are seen as major advantages of non-invasive management. In women treated with the LNG-IUS, this device would be preferred over hysterectomy by 95% of the patients if the expected success rate were >50%.[63]

Endometrial destruction is the second-line treatment for menorrhagia but it can be considered as the first-line treatment for patients in whom other forms of treatment are unsuitable or if the risks relating to surgery are high. The insertion of an LNG-IUS following endometrial resection, to increase the rate of amenorrhoea, may be interesting in some cases.[27] The rationale is that up to 30% of patients need a subsequent procedure which can be avoided by the insertion of an LNG-IUS.

Being an effective contraceptive, together with the strong reduction of MBL, makes it a very attractive method for many women in developed and developing countries. The simple and safe insertion procedure of the Femilis® LNG-IUS could be an added advantage for use by non-specialist providers such as nurses, midwives and general practitioners who are practicing in remote areas as many women lack access to specialized treatment in these areas.

6. Acknowledgment

The authors greatly acknowledge Prof. Dr. G. Van Maele, Dr. Sc. of the Department of Medical Informatics and Statistics, University Hospital Gent, Belgium for providing statistical data analysis for the studies.

Conflict of Interest: Dirk Wildemeersch, MD, PhD, is a Belgian gynaecologist and Medical Director of Contrel Drug Delivery Research, an organization which was established to manage clinical research and to develop and study innovative drug delivery technologies, aimed at finding improved methods for prevention and treatment of gynaecological conditions, improvements to birth control methods, and higher levels of safety, user acceptability, compliance and quality of life for women. Contrel is the manufacturer of

GyneFix®, FibroPlant® and Femilis®. The research organization also provides insertion training for doctors. The funds generated are used for conducting further research and to participate in humanitarian projects.

7. References

[1] Edlund M, Magnuson C, von Schoultz B. Quality of life - a Swedish survey of 2200 women. In: Smith SK, ed. Dysfunctional uterine bleeding. London: Royal Society of Medicine Press, 1994.

[2] Coulter A, Bradlow J, Agass M. Outcomes of referrals to gynaecology outpatient clinics for menstrual problems: an audit of general practice records. Br J Obstet Gynaecol 1991;98;789-796.

[3] Clarke A, Black N. Rowe P, Mott S. Howie K. Indications for and outcomes of total abdominal hysterectomy for benign disease: a prospective cohort study. Br J Obstet Gynaecol 1995;102:611-620.

[4] Cameron IT and Smith SK. Menorrhagia. In: Haemostasis and thrombosis in obstetrics and gynecology. Ed. I Greer, A Turpie and C Forbes. Associated Books, London, 1992, pp. 77-93.

[5] Janssen CA, Scholten PC, Heintz APM. A Simple Visual Assessment Technique to Discriminate Between Menorrhagia and Normal Menstrual Blood Loss. Obstet Gynecol 1995;85,(6):977-982.

[6] World Health Organization. More than half of all pregnant women suffer from anaemia. WHO Presss Release WHO/17, 5 March 1993.

[7] Hurskainen R. Managing drug-resistant essential menorrhagia without hysterectomy. Best Practice &Research Clinical Obstetrics and Gynaecology Vol. 20, No. 5, pp. 681-694, 2006.

[8] Hurskainen R, Teperi J, Rissanen P et al. Clinical outcomes and costs with the levonorgestrel releasing intrauterine system or hysterectomy for treatment of menorrhagia: Randomized trial 5-year follow-up. JAMA: The Journal of the American medical Association 2004; 291: 1456-1463.

[9] Lethaby A, Cooke I, Rees M & Lethaby A. Progesterone or progestogen-releasing intrauterine systems for heavy menstrual bleeding. Cochrane Database of Systematic Reviews 2005; 4: CD002126.

[10] Reid PC & Virtanen-Kari S. Randomised comparative trial of the levonorgestrel intrauterine system and mefenamic acid for the treatment of idiopathic menorrhagia: a multiple analysis using total menstrual fluid loss, menstrual blood loss and pictorial blood loss assessment charts. British Journal of Obstetrics and Gynaecology 2005; 112: 1121-1125.

[11] Wildemeersch D, Schacht E. Treatment of menorrhagia with a novel 'frameless' intrauterine levonorgestrel-releasing drug delivery system, a pilot study. European Journal of Contraception and Reproductive Health Care 2001; 6, 93–101.

[12] Wildemeersch D, Schacht E The effect on menstrual blood loss in women with uterine fibroids of a novel 'frameless' intrauterine levonorgestrel-releasing drug delivery system, a pilot study. European Journal of Obstetrics, Gynecology and Reproductive Biology 2002;102:74-79.

[13] Andrade ATL, Souza JP, Andrade GN, Rowe PJ. Assessment of menstrual blood loss in Brazilian users of the frameless copper-releasing IUD with copper surface are of 330 mm^2 and the frameless levonorgestrel-releasing intrauterine system. Contraception 2004;70:173-7.

[14] Wildemeersch D, Rowe PJ. Assessment of menstrual blood loss in women with idiopathic menorrhagia using the frameless levonorgestrel-releasing intrauterine system. Contraception 2004;70:165-168.

[15] Wildemeersch D, Rowe PJ. Assessment of menstrual blood loss in Belgian users of a new T-shaped levonorgestrel-releasing intrauterine system. Contraception 2005;71:470-473.

[16] Hallberg L, Nilsson L. Determination of menstrual blood loss. Scandinav J Clin Lab Invest 1964;16:244-48.

[17] Shaw ST Jr. On quantifying menstrual blood loss. Contraception 1977;16:283-285.

[18] Newton J, Barnard G, Collins W. A rapid method for measuring menstrual blood loss using automatic extraction. Contraception 1977;16:269-82.

[19] Andrade ATL, Souza JP, Shaw ST Jr, Belsey EM, Rowe PJ. Menstrual blood loss and body iron stores in Brazilian women. Contraception 1991;43:241-49.

[20] Silverberg SG, Haukkamaa M, Arko H, Nilsson CG, Luukkainen T. Endometrial morphology during long-term use of levonorgestrel-releasing intrauterine devices. Int J Gynecol Pathol 1986;5:235-241.

[21] Jones RL, Critchly HO. Morphological and functional changes in the endometrium following intrauterine levonorgestrel delivery. Hum Reprod 2000;15 (suppl 3):162-72.

[22] Rutanen E-M. Insulin-like growth factors and insulin-like growth factors binding proteins in the endometrium: effect of intrauterine levonorgestrel delivery. Hum Reprod 2000;15 (suppl 3):173-81.

[23] Haliloglu B, Celik A, Ilter E, Bozkurt S, Ozekici U Comparison of uterine artery blood flow with levonorgestrel intrauterine system and copper intrauterine device. Contraception 83 (2011) 578-81.

[24] Nath Roy S, Bhattacharya S. Benefits and risks of pharmacological agents used for the treatment of menorrhagia. Drug Safety 2004;27:75-90.

[25] Milson I, Andersson K, Andresch B, Rybo G. A comparison of flurbiprofen, tranexamic acid and a levonorgestrel intrauterine contraceptive device in the treatment of idiopathic menorrhagia. Am J Obstet Gynecol 1991;164:879-83.

[26] Kaunitz AM, Meredith S, Inki P, Kubba A, Sanchez-Ramos L. Levonorgestrel-Releasing Intrauterine System and Endometrial Ablation in Heavy Menstrual Bleeding. A Systematic Review and Meta-Analysis. Obstet Gynecol 2009; 113: 1103-16.

[27] Maia H Jr, Maltez A, Coelho G, Athayde C, Coutinho EM. Insertion of mirena after endometrial resection in patients with adenomyosis. J Am Assoc Gynecol Laparosc. 2003; 10:512-6.

[28] Altman D, Granath F, Cnattingius S, Falconer C. Hysterectomy and risk of stress-uriniary-incontinence. The Lancet 2007; 370:1494-1499. BMJ 2010;341: c3929doi: 10.1136/bmj.c3929.

[29] Hurskainen R, Teperi J, Rissanen P, Aalto AM, Grenman S, Kivelä A, Kujansuu E, Vuorma S, Yliskoski M, Paavonen J. Clinical outcomes and costs with the levonorgestrel-releasing intrauterine system or hysterectomy for treatment of menorrhagia. JAMA 2004;291:1456-63.

[30] Majorbanks J, Lethaby A, Farquhar C. Surgery versus medical therapy for heavy menstrual bleeding. Cochrane Database System Review 2003;(2):CD003855.
[31] Lukes AS, Kadir RA, Peyvandi F, Kouides PA. Disorders of hemostasis and excessive menstrual bleeding: prevalence and clinical impact. Fertil Steril 2005;84:1338-44.
[32] Munro MG, Lukes AS for the Abnormal Uterine Bleeding and Underlying Hemostatic Disorders Consensus Group: Abnormal uterine bleeding and underlying hemostatic disorders: report of a consensus process. Fertil Steril 2005;84:1335-7.
[33] Chi C, Huq FY, Kadir RA. Levonorgestrel-releasing intrauterine system for the management of heavy menstrual bleeding in women with inherited bleeding disorders: long-term follow-up. Contraception 83 (2011) 242-7.
[34] Kadir RA, Chi C. Levonorgestrel intrauterine system: bleeding disorders and anticoagulant therapy. Contraception 75 (2007) S123-S129.
[35] Chi C, Pollard D, Tuddenham EGD, Kadir RA. Menorrhagia in Adolescents with Inherited Bleeding Disorders. J Pediatr Adolesc Gynecol 2010;23:215-22.
[36] Grimes DA, Hubacher D, Lopez LM, Schulz KF. Non-steroidal anti-inflammatory drugs for heavy bleeding or pain associated with intrauterine-device use. Cochrane Database Syst Rev 2006;(4):CD006034.
[37] Hubacher D. Preventing copper IUD removals due to side effects among first time users: placebo-controlled randomized controlled trial to study the effect of prophylactic ibuprofen. Hum Reprod 2007;21:1467-72.
[38] Benacerraf BR, Shipp TD, Bromly B. Three-dimensional ultrasound detection of abnormally located intrauterine contraceptive devices which are the source of pelvic pain and abnormal bleeding. Ultrasound Obstet Gynecol 2009; 34: 110-5.
[39] Shipp TD, Bromly B. Benacerraf BR. The width of the uterine cavity is narrower in patients with an embedded intrauterine device (IUD) compared to a normally positioned IUD. J Ultrasound Med 2010; 29: 1453-6.
[40] Wildemeersch D, Rowe PJ. Assessment of menstrual blood loss in Belgian users of the frameless copper-releasing IUD with copper surface area of 200 mm2 and users of a copperlevonorgestrel-releasing intrauterine system. Contraception 2004;70: 169-72.
[41] Wildemeersch D, Rowe PJ. Assessment of menstrual blood loss in women with idiopathic menorrhagia using the frameless levonorgestrel-releasing intrauterine system. Contraception 2004; 70: 165-8.
[42] Milsom I, Andersson K, Jonasson K, Lindstedt G, Rybo G. The influence of the Gyne-T 380s IUD on menstrual blood Loss and iron status. Contraception 1995; 52: 175-9.
[43] Kivijarvi A, Timoneb H, Rajamaki A, Gronroos M. Iron deficiency in women using copper intrauterine devices. Obstet Gynecol 1986; 67: 95-8.
[44] Hallberg L, Högdahl AH, Nilsson L, Rybo G. Menstrual blood loss, a population study. Acta Obstet Gynec Scand 1966;45:320-51.
[45] Guillebaud J, Bonnar J, Morehead J, Mathews A. Menstrual blood loss with intrauterine devices. Lancet 1976;21:387-90.
[46] Jacobs A, Butler EB. MBL in iron deficiency anemia. The Lancet 1965;11:407-9.
[47] Nisolle M and Donnez J. Medical management of uterine fibroids: short-term therapy with GnRH agonists. In: Brosens I, Lunenfeld B, Donnez J, eds. Pathogenesis and medical management of uterine fibroids. Carnforth, UK: Parthenon Publishing, 1999:113-119.

[48] Donnez J, Gillerot S, Squifflet J and Nisolle M. Progestogens and antiprogestogens. In: Brosens I, Lunenfeld B, Donnez J, eds. Pathogenesis and medical management of uterine fibroids. Carnforth, UK: Parthenon Publishing, 1999:121-128.
[49] Assakis VJ, Jordan VC. Gynecological effects of tamoxifen and the association with breast carcinoma. Int J Gynecol Obstet.1995, 49:241-257.
[50] Grigorieva V. Chen-Mok M, Tarasova M, et al. Use of a levonorgestrel-releasing intrauterine system to treat bleeding related to uterine leiomyomas. Fert Steril 2003;79:1194-8.
[51] Mercorio F, De Simone R, Di Spiezio Sardo A, et al. The effect of a levonorgestrel-releasing intrauterine device in the treatment of myoma-related menorrhagia. Contraception 2003;67:277-80.
[52] MagalhÃ£es J, Aldrighi JM, de Lima GR: Uterine volume and menstrual patterns in users of the levonorgestrel-releasing intrauterine system with idiopathic menorrhagia or menorrhagia due to leiomyomas. Contraception; 2007;75:193-8.
[53] Inki P, Hurskainen R. Palo P, et al. Comparison of ovarian cyst formation in women using the levonorgestrel-releasing intrauterine system vs. hysterectomy. Ultrasound Obstet Gynecol 2002;20:381-85.
[54] Maruo T, Matsuo H, Shimomura Y. et al. Effects of progesterone on growth factor expression in human uterine leiomyoma. Steroids 3003;68:817-24.
[55] Wildemeersch D, Schacht E, Wildemeersch P. Treatment of primary and secondary dysmenorrrhoea with a novel "frameless" intrauterine levonorgestrel-releasing drug delivery system: a pilot study. Eur J Contracept & Reprod Health Care 2001;6:192-198.
[56] Cohen BJ, Gibor Y. Anemia and menstrual blood loss. Obstet Gynecol Surv 1980;35:597-618.
[57] Wood C. Menorrhagia: a management update. Modern Medicine of Australia 1999;42:65-75.
[58] Hurskainen R. Managing drug-resistant essential menorrhagia without hysterectomy. Best Practice &Research Clinical Obstetrics and Gynaecology Vol. 20, No. 5, pp. 681-694, 2006.
[59] National Institute Clinical Excellence (NICE, UK).[59] New guidelines on heavy menstrual bleeding. Issue 05: 5 mar 2007 (www.nice.org.uk/cg044).
[60] Bahamondes L, Petta CA, Fernandes A, Monteiro I. Use of the levonorgestrel-releasing intrauterine system in women with endometriosis, chronic pelvic pain and dysmenorrheal. Contraception 75 (2007) S134–S139.
[61] Fedele L, Bianci S, Raffaelli R, Portuese A, Dorta M. Treatment of adenomyosis-associated menorrhagia with a levonorgestrel-releasing intrauterine device. Fertil Steril. 1997 Sep;68(3):426-429.
[62] Wildemeersch D, Pylyser K, De Wever N, Dhont M. Treatment of non atypical and atypical endometrial hyperplasia with a levonorgestrel-releasing intrauterine system: long-term follow-up. Maturitas 57 (2007) 210–213.
[63] Boudrez P, Bongers MY, Mol BWJ. Treatment of dysfunctional uterine bleeding: patient preferences for endometrial ablation, a levonorgestrel-releasing intrauterine device, or hysterectomy. Fert Steril 2004;82:160-166.

7

Amenorrhea and Endometrial Ablation: A Review and New Insights

Immerzeel Peter and Van Eijndhoven Hugo
Isala Klinieken Zwolle
Netherlands

1. Introduction

Amenorrhea and menorrhagia are opposites and not in any way related to each other. However, the main goal of endometrial ablative therapy in menorrhagia is to establish amenorrhea. Therefore, it is obvious that we spend some words on this subject. Menorrhagia is an important problem in premenopausal women visiting their gynaecologist or general practitioner. Treatment of menorrhagia is diverse: oral contraceptives, intra-uterine hormone devices, hysterectomy, or, endometrial ablation. The latter has proved itself as a valuable technique which is fast, minimal invasive and cost-effective without need for hospitalisation. In this chapter we will discuss the history, the different techniques, indications and complications and some special features of endometrial ablation.

2. History

Heavy menstrual bleeding or menorrhagia affects approximately 20% of all healthy premenopausal women aged 30-49 (Vessey, 1992), causing anaemia and/or a decrease in quality of life. It is a widespread problem and approximately 12% of all referrals to a gynaecologist are related to heavy menstrual bleeding.

First step in treatment is medical therapy, that is to say oral contraceptives. The efficiency of this therapy is variable and the best result with an optimal medicamental treatment is about 50% reduction of the amount of blood loss (EHC, 1992). The levonorgestrel-releasing intrauterine system is more effective and reduces heavy menstrual bleeding in 94% (Irvine, 1998). However, many women prefer a non-hormonal treatment when the conservative treatment with oral contraceptives or a levonorgestrel-releasing system is not sufficient. In this group of patients sometimes surgical therapy is indicated. For decades hysterectomy was the only surgical treatment. Although very effective, hysterectomy involves significant physical implications, a high price in both social and economic costs, a high rate of major and minor post-operative complications and a long recovery time.

Targeted endometrial destruction was originally developed and published in 1936 by Bardenheuer (Bardenheuer, 1937), using a radiofrequency electrosurgical probe passing through the cervical canal into the endometrial cavity without endoscopic guidance. Another technique, was developed in 1967 by Cahan and Brockunier (Cahan and

Brockunier, 1967), called cryoendometrial ablation. They used a probe, also without endoscopic guidance, cooling the endometrial lining. Both techniques did not become widely adopted and the use of endometrial ablation was limited until the introduction of hysteroscopy. After 1980, a new less invasive, uterine sparing method, the hysteroscopic endometrial ablation was developed. The first techniques described were the laser ablation, transcervical endometrial resection (TCRE) and rollerball endometrial ablation. The aim of all three techniques was to remove, or destroy the entire thickness of the uterine endometrial lining and the basal endometrial glands present in the superficial myometrium. These techniques were all hysteroscopic, performed under general anaesthesia and requiring good surgical skills for the best therapeutic effect. These techniques, referred as the first generation, are intensively studied and became the gold standard for endometrial ablation in treatment of heavy menstrual bleeding. Compared to medicamental treatment the results of these techniques were much better but obviously less effective than hysterectomy. However, patient satisfaction is high and complication rate is lower compared to hysterectomy (Abbot, 2002).
With ongoing development, a new generation of minimal invasive techniques without the need of the typical surgical skills of the first generation, was born: the so called second generation endometrial ablation. The main difference between the first and second generation techniques is the absence of the hysteroscopy. This makes the technique easier to perform, with a lower risk of complications and without the need for skilled surgeons. Although a whole number of methods are taken together and called the second generation, in reality it is a wide variety of different techniques: the hot liquid balloons, the microwave, bipolar ablation, phototherapy and chemical destruction of the endometrial lining. With the development of the second generation, operation time and hospitalisation became shorter, with a lower need for complimentary surgery following non satisfactory treatment and a higher satisfactory rate (Lethaby, 2009).

3. Endometrial ablation techniques

The development of endometrial destruction techniques starts around 1937 as mentioned before. For long time the idea of endometrial destruction was leaved. During the eighties of previous century, the idea was revived due to new techniques and insights from other medical specialities, especially the urologists.After that period the development of the techniques was a bit faster and is going on till today. Table 1. summarizes the available techniques.

3.1 First generation techniques

3.1.1 Laser

In 1981 Milton Goldrath introduced the first hysteroscopically assisted photo vaporisation of the endometrium (Goldrath, 1981). They used a device that could be introduced through the instrument channel of an operating hysteroscope. The method he used was a Neodymium: Yttrium Alumnum Garnet laser, (Nd:YAG). Because of the high costs and the development of new hysteroscopic techniques, gynaecologists collectively replaced the heavy and expensive technique of laser ablation by the resectoscope. These newer methods, influenced by the resectoscope of the urologist, were adopted worldwide.

Endometrial destruction techniques.
Hysteroscopic: • Nd:YAG laser • Electorsurgical rollerbal • Transcervical resection.

Non hysteroscopic:
• Balloon thermal ablation
  • CavatermTM plus
  • Thermachoice®
  • Thermablate®
  • Menotreat®
• Free fluid thermal ablation
  • Hydro Thermablate®
• Microwave ablation
  • MEA®
• Bipolar radiofrequency ablation
  • Novasure®
• Cryotherapy
  • HerOption®

Other: • Endometrial laser intrauterine thermal therapy: ELITT   • Gynelease® • Chemoablation • Photodynamic ablation

Table 1. Endometrial destruction techniques.

3.1.2 Electrosurgical rollerball and transcervical resection of the endometrium

Inspired by the results and knowledge of the urologic resections, new techniques were invented to replace the laser photo vaporisation of the endometrium. The resectoscope that was developed could pass through the instrument channel of an operating hysteroscope. With this loop shaped monopolar electro coagulating assisted resectoscope endometrium can be removed from the entire endometrial cavity (Decherney, 1987). The electrosurgical rollerball is also a hysteroscopic monopolar technique, with the difference that it is not resecting, but only coagulating the endometrial lining. Both methods could be and are often combined in the same session.

3.2 Second generation techniques

The difficulties experienced with the first generation paved the way to develop new techniques without a need for typical surgical skills and without the complications associated with the hysteroscopic technique. Although these newer methods do not require direct visualisation of the endometrium by hysteroscopy, they are mutually different, using either heat or cold, microwave or radiofrequency energy. Compared to the first generation the complication rates are lower, operation time is shorter and some of these techniques can be applied in an outpatient setting. Their effectiveness and safety are intensively studied and compared to the first generation techniques. These randomised controlled trials are summarized at the end of this paragraph.

3.2.1 Balloon thermal ablation

Balloon thermal ablation basically is a technique in which a balloon catheter attached to a central unit is placed in the uterine cavity. The balloon is then filled with a distension fluid and because of a constant pressure the balloon shapes the endometrial cavity as effective as possible. By heating and circulating the fluid for a specific time, endometrial ablation is accomplished . The balloon techniques differ in cervical dilatation, distension fluid, temperature of fluid, distension pressure and operating time. The main complications are postoperative nausea and uterine cramps, probably related to uterine distension and prostaglandin release. All available techniques are listed below.

3.2.1.1 Cavaterm™ plus

The original Cavaterm™plus unit, consists of a computerised central unit and a single-use silicone balloon. The balloon size can be adjusted according to the size of the uterine cavity. The fluid used is 1.5% glycine, heated from the centre of the catheter to 75 degrees Celsius and constantly circulated throughout the system via a pump. The system monitors the pressure within the circuit and it is maintained between 220-240 mm Hg. The treatment time is 15 minutes and the depth of endometrial ablation is 6-8 mm. Cavaterm plus system uses a 5% dextrose solution and requires cervical dilatation only to 6 mm. The duration of treatment is 10 minutes and there is no need for pre-treatment of the endometrium. The device is portable and has a small diameter probe. To be effective, the intimate contact between the balloon and the endometrium is important. Patient satisfaction rate as recorded is 83% after two years, amenorrhea was achieved in 39% of the patients. (El Thouky, 2004).

3.2.1.2 Thermachoice III

Thermachoice ® comprises a single use balloon catheter, a connecting cable and a dedicated controller unit that is powered from a standard alternating current wall outlet. The outside diameter of the catheter is 5.5 mm and the heating element is incorporated in the balloon itself. After exposure of the cervix and the required dilation, the balloon-tipped catheter is passed through the cervical canal into the endometrial cavity. The surgeon uses a syringe to inflate the balloon with 5% dextrose and water to a predetermined pressure of 160 tot 180 mm Hg. The dedicated controller unit is then activated, therby heating the element and the fluid. The target balloon temperature is 87 degrees Celsius and ablation time is about 8 minutes. The depth of ablation is 4.5 mm. Patient satisfaction rate as registered is 95.9% after one year, amenorrhea is achieved in 15.2% of the patients, complimentory surgery was necessary in 33% of the patients after 5 years (Loffer, 2002).

3.2.1.3 Thermablate®

Thermablate®, an endometrial ablation system (EAS), consists of a light weight, reusable, hand-held treatment control unit with a single-use disposable catheter of 6 mm in diameter. Following insertion of the prelubricated balloon into the endometrial cavity, a glycerine solution is heated to 173 degrees Celsius and the pressure is automatically maintained at 180 mm Hg for a treatment cycle of 2 minutes and 8 seconds. Tissue necrosis to a uniform depth of 4-5 mm. can be accomplished.

3.2.1.4 Menotreat ®

MenoTreat® is a relatively new method, which is mainly used in the Scandinavian countries. The system consists of a disposable silicone catheter with a balloon (two possible sizes) and a control unit. The cervix is dilated to 8 mm for insertion of the 7 mm diameter catheter. The fluid, saline is heated to 85 degrees Celsius in the control unit and circulates from there through the catheter. The pressure is maintained at 200 mm Hg and the treatment time is 11 minutes.

3.2.2 Free fluid endometrial ablation

Endometrial ablation with HydroThermablator® (HTA) is based on the principle of circulating heated free fluid and is the only technique with hysteroscopic monitoring during the procedure. The device consists of a single use 7.8-mm sheath which is connected to a proprietary controller unit. The controller unit regulates the processes of uterine distension, creation of a closed circuit, fluid heating, and monitoring of temperature and circuit volume. The distending medium is normal saline drawn from a bag mounted on a attached, modified IV pole. After dilatation of the cervix and priming of the circuit, the telescope and sheath are placed transcervical into the endometrial cavity. After confirmation of intracavitary positioning, the microprocessor-controlled automated system is started. The tip of the endoscope and sheath are held at the level of the internal cervical OS. The process takes approximately 3 minutes to heat the fluid to 90 degrees Celsius. The hot fluid is maintained for10 minutes in the uterine cavity, after which it is allowed to cool down in one minute before removal of the device. Necrosis depth is about 3-4 mm. The process can be stopped at any time by the surgeon. If there is a loss of more than 10 mL of the distending medium either through the cervix or the fallopian tubes, the system stops the procedure automatically. To prevent leakage of hot fluid through the fallopian tubes the intra uterine pressure is kept below 55 mm Hg. Specific complications of this technique are perineal, vaginal and thigh burns when the hot fluid leaks from the cervix. The amenorrhea rate reported with the HydroThermablator was 53%, with decrease in menstrual bleeding in 94% of the patients treated. Patient satisfaction rate is high, 98% after 3 years and complementary surgery is necessary in about 11% of the patients (Goldrath, 2003).

3.2.3 Microwave endometrial ablation

There are two versions of the microwave endometrial ablation (MEA) device, one reusable and the other disposable. FemWave® comprises an 8 mm outside diameter probe attached through a reusable cable to a dedicated control module. The microwave frequency is 9.2 GHz, power output 30 W, and the local tissue is heated to about 90 degrees Celsius, achieving a depth of tissue necrosis of about 5-6 mm. The probe also contains an integrated thermal coupling device that transmits information about adjacent tissue temperature to the control module. Activation and control of the device is entirely in the hands of the surgeon. Once the cervix is dilated, hysteroscopic imaging confirms intracavitary placement and after both the canal and cavity are confirmed to be intact, the microwave probe is inserted to the uterine fundus. When the measured temperature of the tissue around the probe reaches 30 degrees Celsius, the device is activated and the surgeon uses sweeping movements in the horizontal plane until a treatment temperature threshold of 80 degrees Celsius is reached. By gradually withdrawing the device the surgeon covers the entire endometrial surface. When the tip of the probe reaches the area that approximates the location of the cervical channel, the device is deactivated and the probe is removed. Treatment time depends on cavity size and is usually about 2-4 minutes. Endometrial curettage prior to MEA application is not recommended as it increases the risk of unrecognised uterine perforation and subsequent microwave-induced bowel damage. Patient satisfaction after 5 years is about 71%, and amenorrhea is achieved in 84% of patients after 5 years (Sambrook, 2010).

3.2.4 Radiofrequency endometrial ablation

NovaSure® is an ablation technique that uses impedance controlled bipolar radiofrequency (RF) for endometrial ablation. The system is based on a dedicated microprocessor-based control unit and a single use 7.2 outside diameter probe with a bipolar gold mesh electrode array located at the distal end. To detect a perforation of the myometrium, the probe contains a system for determining the integrity of the endometrial cavity based on injection of a fixed volume of CO2. After appropriate cervical dilatation, the electrode assembly is inserted transcervically and the electrode is deployed by retraction of an outer sleeve. The electrodes have a triangular shape that correspond with the surface of the uterine cavity. The surgeon then measures the intercornual distance using an indicator on the probe and enters this value together with the cavity length into the controller unit allowing the system to calculate the amount of power required. Before activation, the dedicated controller unit performs a so called uterine integrity test to exclude a perforation. After this RF energy is applied to the endometrial tissue and at the same time steam and carbonized debris is evacuated from the uterine cavity. This process results in electrosurgical vaporization and underlying desiccation in a relatively short time (90-120 seconds). The depth of vaporization and desiccation varies throughout the uterine cavity, less in the cornual areas and more in the other areas. The process is controlled by increasing tissue impedance of the adjacent desiccated tissue, shutting the system off when it exceeds 50 omega. Patient satisfaction rate of the Novasure® method is 92.8%. After one year, 41% of the patients reported amenorrhea and 88.3% with a satisfactory decrease in monthly menstrual bleeding. Complementary surgery is seen in 9.8% of patients after 5 years (Kleijn, 2008).

3.2.5 Cryotherapy

Cryotherapy was first used in 1967 but enthusiasm was restrained by reports of pelvic abscesses after this procedure. With the development of transcervical uterus sparing techniques for endometrial ablation, the principle of cryotherapy was revitalized resulting in a device called Her Option®. Destruction of the endometrium is achieved by freezing it to -90 degrees Celsius. The device consists of a disposable 4.5 mm outside diameter probe attached to a handle and cable, which is connected to a dedicated controller unit. After exposure of the cervix, cervical dilation is performed if necessary, and the device is inserted into the uterine cavity. The surgeon activates the controller which super cools the tip of the probe to -90 degrees Celsius, resulting in a progressively expanding elliptical frozen zone involving both endometrium and myometrium. The size of this zone depends on the exposure time and can be monitored by the surgeon using transabdominal ultrasound. To cover all the endometrium usually 2 or 3 cycles, with a total treatment time of about 10 minutes, are necessary. The depth of tissue necrosis is about 12 mm. Clinical outcomes shows a reduction in menstrual bleeding of 84.6%, with amenorrhea rates not well documented. Long term follow up shows a hysterectomy rate of about 7% and a reablation rate of 8.1% after 24 months (Townsend, 2003).

3.2.6 Endometrial laser intrauterine thermal therapy (ELITT)

The ELITT diode laser system (Gynelase®) is a system that produces 830nm diode laser light through a flexible quartz fibre to an intrauterine device., This device is composed of three fibres that ensure circumferential diffusion of the active laser light inside the uterine cavity. The fibres adhere to the uterine walls and uniformly distribute the laser beam over the endometrium from the fundus to the isthmus of the uterine cavity. This procedure exploits the thermic and coagulative properties of the laser beam in a way that the poorly accessible cornual endometrium also can be ablated. The cervical canal is first dilated up to 7 mm, and the closed diffuser device is then introduced into the uterine cavity. When it reaches the fundus, the surgeon opens the lateral fibres, giving the system an inverted triangular shape that adapts to the uterine cavity. The laser is activated for 7 minutes in a continuous tissue exposure mode in three consecutive steps; distension fluid is not required for this procedure. Results of ELITT show an amenorrhea rate of 61% after 36 months and an overall patient satisfactory rate of 89%, re-intervention by hysterectomy is reported in 5% of the patients (Perino, 2004).

3.2.7 Photodynamic therapy

Photodynamic therapy for endometrial ablation (PEA), provides a photo oxidation-based, selective endometrial destruction, tested mainly in animal studies. There is only one human feasibility study executed (Degen, 2004). PEA was performed by injecting 5-aminolevulinic acid (ALA) into the uterine cavity. After three to six hours a light dose of 160J/cm3 at a wavelength of 635 nm was applied to the endometrial lining using a balloon-light diffuser. The light was fractionated in sequences of 5 minutes of illumination followed by gaps of 2 minutes. Bleeding patterns were significantly reduced 1-3 months after treatment, but this reduction was not significant after long term follow up. This technique is still in an experimental stage.

3.2.8 Chemoablation

With so called chemo ablation 95% trichloroacetate (TCA) is used to destroy the endometrium. This compound is also used in the treatment of papilloma warts. Before the procedure, patients receive non-steroidal anti-inflammatory drugs orally. Under local anaesthesia, with a paracervical block, a 3mm cannula must be inserted into the cervix. Through this cannula the volume of TCA needed is instilled into the uterine cavity. Leakage from the cervix is collected in a sponge. The treatment results were recorded both with and without pre-treatment with a GnRH analogue one month before surgery. Patient satisfactory after 1 year is 93.3% and 95.6%, respectively in the group without and with pre-treatment. Amenorrhea is accomplished in 31.1% and 26.7% in these groups and reduction of bleeding is reported in 68.9 and 66.7%, respectively (Kucuk, 2005).

4. Randomized controlled trials

Many studies have been performed over the last years, involving both first and second generation techniques. We have selected the most relevant randomized controlled trials with long term follow-up. The results are summarized in table with regard to patients satisfactory, amenorrhea rates, reintervention surgery rates and the main conclusions of the authors.

Study	Satisfactory	Amenorrhea Rate	Reintervention surgery	Conclusion
Studies comparing 1st generation techniques with 2nd generation techniques.				
Sambrook, 2009 10 year follow up: - MEA - TCRE	60% 52%	83% 88%	17% 28%	Both techniques achieve significant and comparable improvement in menstrual symptoms, health-related quality of life and high rates of satisfaction. With the known operative advantages, lower costs and fewer hysterectomies, it is clear that MEA is a more effective and efficient treatment for heavy menstrual loss than TCRE.
Goldrath, 2003 - HTA - Rollerball ablation	98% 97%	53% 46%		Endometrial ablation with the HTA is a safe, effective, and durable treatment of menorrhagia in a broad patient population. It offers advantages over RB by reducing anaesthesia requirements, reducing operating time, and eliminating risks of excessive fluid absorption, and is more easily learned.
Studies comparing 2nd generation with 2nd generation techniques				
Kleijn, 2008 5 year follow up. - Bipolar radiofrequency. - Thermal balloon		48% 32%	9.8% 12.6%	At 5 years follow up, bipolar thermal ablation was superior over balloon ablation in the treatment of menorrhagia.
Sambrook, 2009, - MEA - Thermal balloon	76% 77%	41% 38%		Both treatments are acceptable to women, with high levels of satisfaction. Microwave is quicker to perform with faster hospital discharge.

Table 2. Randomized controlled trials performed last years.

A large Cochrane Database review intensively studied and combined the studies comparing first and second generation techniques (Lethaby, 2009). The authors conclude that endometrial ablation offer a less invasive surgical alternative to hysterectomy. The conclusions of this review slightly favour the second generation techniques. Advantages were a shorter surgery time (15minutes), the use of local anaesthesia, and fewer complications like fluid overload, uterine perforation, cervical lacerations and haematometra. However, the second generation was associated with more equipment failure and patients were more likely to suffer from nausea, vomiting and uterine cramping postoperatively.

4.1 Conclusion

Main problem in comparing the first and second generation techniques is the heterogeneity of all studies. Especially, in the first generation, experience and skills of the surgeon are important cofounding factors. No significant differences are found in amenorrhoea rates and requirement for any additional surgery or hysterectomy between both generations. In general, one can say that with the introduction of the second generation the operation time is shorter, complications like fluid overload and perforation are reduced and the skills and experience of the surgeon has become less important.

5. Factors affecting outcome of endometrial ablation

The outcome of endometrial ablation regarding patients' satisfaction , amenorrhea rates and side effects, is intensively studied. In this paragraph we will discuss the factors that possibly affect the outcome of endometrial ablation.

5.1 Patient factors

Patient characteristics are important to decide whether a treatment modality is suitable for an individual patient. There are not many studies reporting pre operative factors influencing the outcome of global endometrial ablation. Patient factors that could predict amenorrhea after endometrial ablation are: an age older than 45 years, uterine length less than nine centimetres and endometrial thickness less than four millimetres (El-Nashar, 2009). Patient factors found to be prognostic for treatment failure are an age younger than 45 years, parity of five or greater, prior tubal ligation and history of dysmenorrhoea (El-Nashar, 2009). The role of leiomyomas in the outcome of endometrial ablation has not been established. Submucous leiomyomas increase the volume of menstrual bleeding by mechanisms that are, to date, not well understood. One of these mechanisms is probably the larger cross sectional area of endometrium of the uterine cavity. As a result, endometrial ablation is assumed to be successful in the treatment of women with myomas, but on the other hand, leiomyomas are also considered an important reason for treatment failure. Literature on this subject is not conclusive, and the presences of myomas has often been reason for exclusion. With the development of different new techniques it is expected that the presence of leiomyomas will not always be an exclusion factor for endometrial ablation, e.g. no evidence is found that the presence of leiomyomas is a predictive value for post operative amenorrhea rate or treatment failure (El-Nashar, 2009).

5.2 Preoperative thinning of the endometrium

Complete endometrial destruction is one of the most important determinants of treatment success. During the menstrual cycle endometrial thickness varies from as little as 1mm in the immediate postmenstrual phase to 10 mm or more in the late secretory phase. The techniques described have an ablation depth, ranging mostly from 4-6 mm. It is obvious that an endometrial thickness of 10 mm with a technique infiltration depth of 6 mm, is less effective. Therefore, thinning of the endometrium and planning of the surgery could contribute to a successful outcome. On the other hand, does pre-treatment with agents like GnRH analogues or Danazol add additional side effects and costs to any endometrial ablation procedure? A large Cochrane review was published in 2009. In this study the effect of pre-operative endometrial thinning before endometrial ablation was investigated. (Sowter, 2009).

5.2.1 Gonadotrophin-releasing hormones analogues

Down regulation of the receptors by Gonadotrophin- Releasing Hormones (GnRH) analogues results in a hypoestrogenic state leading to atrophic endometrium. Side effects of the treatment may be hot flushes, vaginal dryness, mood swings, headache, libido loss, difficulties in sleeping and weight changes. The use of GnRH analogues preoperatively showed a significant reduction in endometrial thickness on ultrasound and atrophic endometrial glands on histological examination (Donnez, 1997), This effect of GnRH analogues is larger compared to the effect of Danazol or preoperative admission of progestagens. Comparing hysteroscopic resection of the endometrium with or without GnRH, pre-treatment favours shorter duration of surgery, the surgery was easier to perform and a higher rate of amenorrhea 12 months postoperatively. There is no evidence that these results may be the same in patients treated with the second generation endometrial ablation techniques. Overall, the long-term effects of GnRH analogues as pre-treatment are unclear. (Sowter, 2009).

5.2.2 Danazol

Danazol is a testosterone analogue, with anti-hormonal effect, resulting in a secondary decrease of LH and FSH with ovarian failure. Side effects are acne, greasy skin, stem changes, weight gain, libido loss. Danazol is more effective than no treatment in inducing atrophy in endometrial glands and reducing endometrial thickness as measured with ultrasound. Pre-treatment with Danazol does not lead to higher rate of amenorrhea, patient satisfaction or less women requiring further surgery, under patients undergoing first generation endometrial ablation or resection. Compared to the GnRH analogues, the effect of Danazol on thinning the endometrial lining is inferior. (Sowter, 2009).

5.2.3 Progestagens

Pre-treatment with progestagens does not lead to an adequate reduction of endometrial thickness or atrophy of the endometrial glands (Rich, 1995). The use of progestagens is not recommended at all pre-operatively except in case of a trial (Sowter, 2009).

5.3 Surgical skills

One of the reasons for the development of the second generation techniques are the long learning curve and advanced surgical skills necessary for an adequate hysteroscopic resection of the endometrium. It is demonstrated that complication risk and treatment failure of the first generation techniques are much higher when the experience of the surgeon is limited to less than 100 procedures. (Overton, 1997). With the introduction of the second generation, the advanced operating skills have become less important without impairing treatment results or patients satisfaction (Lethaby, 2009).

5.4 Conclusion

Although pre-treatment with both GnRH analogues and Danazol results in thinning of the endometrial layer, they do not seem to offer any benefit regarding to treatment outcome, patients satisfaction or number of complications. The experience and surgical skills of the surgeon are important factors in the first generation hysteroscopic techniques. Specially, the presence of large myomas, the size of the uterus and the endometrial thickness seem to be a limitation for the use of the second generation techniques

6. Complications

With the development of first and second generation endometrial ablative techniques for treating heavy menstrual bleeding, its use expanded really fast during the last decades. Advantages of these therapy compared to hysterectomy are the shorter operation time, the shorter post operative period, the cost effectiveness and the lower morbidity and mortality compared to hysterectomy . However, both peri- and postoperative complications related to endometrial ablation are described.

6.1 Perioperative complications

Perioperative complications are strongly related to the experience of the surgeon and the technique used. In general, second generation techniques have a lower complication rate due to shorter operating time and compared to the hysteroscopic assisted methods relatively easy procedures. In the Mistletoe study (Overton, 1997), complications of more than 10000 patients treated in the United Kingdom between 1993 and 1994 with endometrial resection, endometrial ablation by rollerball and laser, cryotherapy and radiofrequency ablation were registered. Most common complications with the first generation techniques are peri- or postoperative haemorrhage and uterine perforation. Haemorrhage was reported in 2.38% of the cases, ranging from 0.97% in case of roller ball alone to 3.53% with the combination of endometrial dissection and rollerball. Uterine perforation was reported in 1.48% of the cases. The experience of the surgeon with the technique used is the most important factor influencing the complication rate (Overton, 1997).

6.2 Postoperative complications

Post operative complications diagnosed after treatment or after discharge from the hospital include heavy bleeding, abdominal pain, urinary retention, hypotension, nausea, vomiting, bradycardia, chest pain, urinary tract infection, haematurie, hyponatraemia, pyrexia, deep venous thrombosis and fluid overload syndrome. These complications are rare and only small numbers are recorded. Overall percentages reported range from 0.77%-2.86% of the cases, depending on the technique used (Overton, 1997). The fluid overload syndrome is a well known and possible fatal complication. Absorption of distension fluid could cause hyponatremia with mild symptoms like nausea, but also serious consequencess like seizures and even death due to cerebral oedema. The incidence of fluid overload syndrome is associated with the duration of surgery. In general, the complications as registered in the Mistletoe study are more likely to occur after the first generation techniques. Complications as nausea, vomiting and uterine cramping are more related to the second generation techniques (Lethaby, 2009).

6.3 Late onset complications

Complications diagnosed more than six weeks postoperatively are endometritis, septicaemia, pneumonia, peritonitis, pulmonary embolism and surgery for bowel repair. This group of complications are recorded in 1.25% of the cases (Overton, 1997). A cervical or lower uterine segment stenosis after endometrial ablation can cause a secondary to bleeding in the uterine cavity. Symptoms are amenorrhea in concert with cyclic lower abdominal or pelvic pain. The complaints usually start months and sometimes years after the procedure. Treatment modalities are cervical dilatation, hysteroscopic drainage or hysterectomy. Tubal sterilisation is a risk factor for hysterectomy after endometrial ablation. Abdominal pain is caused by bleeding from persistent or regenerating cornual endometrium causing a focal cornual hematometra with retrograde bleeding into an occluded fallopian tube. This syndrome is called post ablation tubal sterilisation syndrome (PATSS). The exact incidence of central hematometra and PATSS is unknown but it is estimated around 10% of the patients . (McCausland, 2007).

7. Endometrial ablation and pregnancy

Approximately, one in every five premenopausal women refers to a health care professional because of heavy menstrual bleeding. Because endometrial ablation is not reliable as contraceptive, all these women are at risk to become pregnant after the treatment. In two large studies including more than nine thousand patients the pregnancy rate after ablation was 0.68% (Pugh, 2000; Roy and Mattox, 2002). Obviously, when none of the patients had used contraceptives this percentage should have been higher. Pregnancy after endometrial ablation is associated with a number of complications and is therefore considered to be a contraindication.

The literature on complications during pregnancy is limited to case reports. Miscarriage is reported in 21% of the pregnancies after ablation (Hare, 2005). Although ectopic pregnancies are described it is unclear whether the number is increased after endometrial ablation. With an ongoing pregnancy the risk for pre term delivery (31%), pre term labour (21%), pre term rupture of membranes (17%), intra uterine growth restriction (12%) malpresentations (39%), and pathological placentation (17%) are all increased. The latter is notorious, leading to a wrong implantation of the placenta in the uterine wall with a high rate of hysterectomy after caesarean section (Hare, 2005). Moreover, the diagnosis in these cases is difficult because classical ultrasonsgraphic appearances of this abnormality may not be present after ablation. Therefore, patients should be counselled carefully, an active wish for children must be excluded and additional contraceptive methods are necessary after the endometrial ablation. If a patient becomes pregnant, close follow up is advised with monitoring of growth and placentation.

Because many patients do not prefer oral contraceptives or a levonorgestrel device after endometrial ablation, the procedure is frequently combined with laparoscopic sterilisation. Recently, the first reports of the combined approach of endometrial ablation and hysteroscopic sterilisation are published. These studies demonstrate that hysteroscopic essure® sterilisaton after both radiofrequency and balloon endometrial ablation is feasible and safe. Although it is attractive to combine these minimal invasive procedures a serious concern is the reliability of the hysterosalpingography (HSG) as confirmation of the sterilisation. In about 26% tubal occlusion can not be determined by HSG because of severe uterine synechiae, probably caused by the endometrial ablation (Detollenaere, 2011). Whether or not endometrial ablation can safely be performed after an earlier hysteroscopic sterilisation remains to be established.

8. Endometrial ablation and endometrial cancer

Endometrial carcinoma is the most common gynaecologic malignant disease with a prevalence worldwide of 1/1000. Because an endometrial carcinoma is mostly diagnosed in an early stage , FIGO stage 1 (73%) or stage II (10%) the five year survival rates are high, for both stages 91%. The risk for endometrial carcinoma increases between 50-70 years and is 8- fold higher in postmenopausal women. Approximately 50% of the endometrial cancers occur in women with associated risk factors like unopposed estrogen stimulation, obesity, diabetes mellitus, chronic anovulation, hypertension and histological complex atypical endometrial hyperplasia or adenomatous hyperplasia (Bakarat, 2009). The most frequent first symptom of endometrial cancer is post- menopausal loss of blood. As endometrial ablation is a relatively new therapy with a variety of techniques, data on the incidence of endometrial cancer after endometrial ablation are lacking. Most cases are reported after a first generation technique. It is suggested that the incidence of endometrial cancer after ablation is reduced in case of maximal destruction of the endometrium. However, some evidence suggests that incidence of endometrial cancer is unchanged, after EA with first generation techniques (Neuwrith, 2004). It is unclear whether endometrial cancer originates from islands of regenerated endometrium below the basal layer or from adenomyosis. The diagnosis of this type of malignancy may be delayed after ablation because adhesions or scars could mask the symptoms of the disease. In case of post-menstrual bleeding after ablation ultrasound and hysteroscopy can be difficult to perform because of the anatomical distortion of the uterine cavity. (Jarvela, 2002; Luo, 1999) Theoretically, in patients at risk for standard operative therapy, endometrial ablation could play a role in the treatment of endometrial neoplasia or cancer. Whether this treatment modality is a serious option requires further study.

9. Conclusion

In this chapter we discussed the most commonly used methods for endometrial ablation and gave a historic overview of these techniques. For today the "gold standard" is still transcervical endometrial resection with rollerball ablation throughout the world. However, the second generation techniques are developing fast and it is likely that they will replace the first generation. It is important to continue research to establish optimal endometrial ablative therapy to improve amenorrhoea rates, patients satisfaction and reduce the need for hysterectomy.

10. References

Abbott, J. & Garry, R. The surgical management of menorrhagia. *Human Reproduction Update,* Vol. 8, No. 1, (February, 2002), pp. 68–78, ISSN 13554786.

Barakat, R., Markman, M. & Randall, M.. Principles and Practice of Gynecologic Oncology. 5th ed. Philadelphia, PA: Wolters Kluwer Health/Lippincott Williams & Wilkins; 2009.

Bardenheuer FH. Elektrokoagulation der Uterusschleimhaut zur Behandlung klimakterischer blutungen. *Zentralblatt fur Gynakologie,* Vol. 4, 1937, pp. 209–211.

Cahan, W. & Brockunier, A. Cryosurgery of the uterine cavity. *American Journal of Obstetrics and Gynaecology*. Vol. 99, No. 1, September 1967, pp. 38–153.

DeCherney, A., Diamond, M. & Lavy, G. Endometrial ablation for intractable uterine bleeding: hysteroscopic resection. *Obstetrics and Gynaecology*. Vol. 70, No 4, October 1987, pp. 668–670.

Degen, A,. Gabrech, T., Mosimann, L., Fehr, M., Hornung, R., Schwarz, V., Tadir, Y., Steiner, R., Wagnières, G. & Wyss, P. Photodynamic Endometrial Ablation for the Treatment of Dysfunctional Uterine Bleeding: A Preliminary Report. *Lasers in Surgery and Medicine,* Vol. 34, No.1,, 2004, pp. 1–4.

Detollenaere, R., Vleugels, M. & Van Eijndhoven, H. Combining Novasure endometrium ablation and Essure hysteroscopic sterilization: a feasibility study to evaluate the confirmation tests. *Gynecological Surgery*. Vol. 8, No. 1, February 2011, pp. 59-63, ISSN 16132076.

Effective Healthcare. What are effective ways of treating excessive regular menstrual blood loss in primary and secondary care?. *Effective Health Care Bulletin.* Vol. 9, August 1995, pp.1–14.

Goldrath, M. Evaluation of Hydro-ThermAblator and rollerball endometrial ablation for menorrhagia 3 years after treatment. *Journal of the American Association of Gynecologic Laparoscopists* . Vol. 10, No. 4, November 2003, pp. 505–511.

Goldrath, M., Fuller, T. & Segal, S. Laser photovaporization of endometrium for the treatment of menorrhagia. *American Journal of Obstetrics and Gynaecology*. Vol. 140, No. 1, May 1981, pp. 14–19.

Hare, A. & Olah, S. Pregnanacy following endometrial ablation: a review article. *Journal of obstetrics and gynaecology.* Vol. 25, No. 2, February 2005, pp. 108-114.

Irvine, G.,Campbell-Brown, M., Lumsden, M., Heikkila, A., Walker, J. & Cameron, I.. Randomised comparative trial of the levonorgestrel intrauterine systemand norethisterone for the treatment of idiopathic menorrhagia. *British Journal of Obstetrics & Gynaecology.* Vol. 105, No. 6, June 1998, pp. 592–598.

Jarvela, I., Tekay, A. & Santala, M. Ultrasonographic features following thermal balloon endometrial ablation therapy. *Gynecologic and Obstetric Investigations.* Vol. 54, No. 1, 2002, pp.11–16.

Kleijn, J., Engels, R., Bourdrez, P., Mol, B. & Bongers, M. Five-year follow up of a randomised controlled trial comparing NovaSure and ThermaChoice endometrial ablation. *British Journal of Obstetrics & Gynaecology.* Vol. 115, No. 2, January 2008, pp. 193-198.

Kucuk, M. & Okman, T. Intrauterine instillation of trichloroacetic acid is effective for the treatment of dysfunctional uterine bleeding. *Fertility and Sterility* Vol. 83, No. 1, 2005, pp. 189-194

Lethaby, A. Hickey, M. & Garry, R. Enodmetrial destruction techniques for heavy menstrual bleeding. *Cochrane Database Systematic Review* Vol. 7, No. 4, October 2009, CD001501

Loffer, F. & Grainger D. Five-year follow-up of patients participating in a randomized trial of uterine balloon therapy versus rollerball ablation for treatment of menorrhagia. *Journal of the American Association of Gynaecologic Laparoscopy.* Vol. 9, No. 4, November 2002, pp. 429–435.

Luo, X. Lim, C. & Li, L. Hysteroscopic appearance of the endometrial cavity after microwave endometrial ablation. *Journal of Minimal Invasive Gynaecology.* Vol. 17, No. 1, January - February1999, pp. 30–36.

Neuwirth, R., Loffer, F. & Trenhaile, T. The incidence of endometrial cancer after endometrial ablation in a low-risk population. *Journal of the American Association of Gynaecologic Laparoscopists.* Vol. 11, No. 4, November 2004, pp. 492–494.

Overton, C., Hargreaves, J. & Maresh, M. A national survey of the complications of endometrial destruction for menstrual disorders: the MISTLETOE study. *British Journal of Obstetrics and Gynaecology.* Vol 104, No. 12, December 1997, pp. 1351-1359.

Perino, A., Castelli, A., Cucinella, G., Biondo, A., Pane, A. & Venezia, R. A randomized comparison of endometrial laser intrauterine thermotherapy and hysteroscopic endometrial resection. *Fertility and sterilitiy.* Vol. 82, No. 3, September 2004, pp. 731-734.

Pugh, C., Crane, J. & Hogan, T. Successful intrauterine pregnancy after endometrial ablation. *Journal of the American Association of Gynecologic Laparoscopists* Vol. 7, No. 3, August 2000, pp. 391 - 394.

Rich, A., Manyonda I., Patel, R. & Amias, A. A comparison of the efficacy of danazol, norethisterone, cyproterone acetate and medroxyprogesterone acetate in endometrial thinning prior to ablation: a pilot study. *Gynaecological Endoscopy.* Vol. 4, No. 1, 1995, pp. 59–61, ISSN: 09621091.

Roy, K. & Mattox, J. Advances in endometrial ablation. *Obstetrical & Gynaecological Survey,* Vol. 57, No. 12, December 2002, pp. 789 - 802.

Sambrook, A., Bain, C., Parkin, D. & Cooper, K. A rondomised comparison of microwave endometrial ablation with transcervical resection of the endometrium: follow up at a minimum of 10 years. *British Journal of Obstetrics & Gynaecology.* Vol. 116, No. 8, July 2009, pp. 1033-1037.

Sambrook, A., Jack, S. & Cooper, K. Outpatient microwave endometrial ablation: 5-year follow-up of a randomised controlled trial without endometrial preparation versus standard day surgery with endometrial preparation. *British Journal of Obstetrics & Gynaecology.* Vol.117, No. 4, March 2010, pp.493–496.

Sowter. Pre-operative endometrial thinning agents before endometrial destruction for heavy menstrual bleeding (Review) *Cochrane database systematicreview,* Vol 3, 2009, CD 001124.

Townsend, D., Duleba, A. & Wilkes, M. Durability of treatment effects after endometrial cryoablation versus rollerball electroablation for abnormal uterine bleeding: two-year results of a multicenter randomized trial. *American Journal of Obstetrics and Gynaecology*. Vol. 188, No. 3, March 2003, pp. 699–701.

Vessey, M., Villard-Mackintosh, L., McPherson, K., Coulter, A. & Yeates, D. The epidemiology of hysterectomy: findings in a large cohort study. *British Journal of Obstetrics & Gynaecology*. Vol. 99, No. 5, May 1992, pp.402–407.

8

Recent Clinical Applications of Kampo Medicine in Amenorrhea

Toshiaki Kogure
Department of Japanese Oriental Medicine,
Gunma Central & General hospital, Maebashi City
Japan

1. Introduction

1.1 Japanese herbal (Kampo) medicine in Japan

Japanese Herbal (Kampo) Medicine, which is covered by national health insurance in Japan, is often prescribed in the primary care field, and is also applied as an alternative remedy for several gynecological diseases such as menstrual disorders, and menopausal symptoms. Since ancient times, a wide variety of Kampo formulae have been used traditionally and found to be clinically effective in gynecological diseases. These formulae usually contain components from several medicinal plants that are thought to exert estrogenic effects contributing to the effective treatment of menstrual disorders (1 - 6). The clinical use of traditional herbal medicines in menopausal women has previously been reported (7).

1.2 Characteristics of Japanese herbal (Kampo) medicines

Kampo Medicine has two features that differ from Western Medicine, i) the Kampo formula is composed of crude drugs, not purified chemical products; ii) the diagnostic system in Kampo Medicine is different from that in Western medicine. Kampo formulae are generally composed of several herbal components, therefore it is considered that these remedies are safe. However, pseudoaldosteronism caused by licorice root is a well known adverse effect (8), and there are also allergic effects, such as skin eruptions (9) and liver injury (10), that can be induced by crude preparations. It is also thought that Kampo diagnosis may not be easy for readers to understand. When we treat the patients with menstrual disorders with Kampo Medicine, it is necessary to establish a Kampo diagnosis as well as a diagnosis by Western medicine. This issue makes it difficult to perform controlled clinical trials. Therefore, there is very little evidence supporting the use of Kampo formulae for gynecological diseases, although Kampo formulae are often prescribed for gynecological diseases in Japan.
In this chapter, we describe estrogen-like activities and clinical effects on menstrual disorders, as well as current topics concerning Kampo therapeutic strategy for menstrual disorders.

2. Action on the hypothalamus-pituitary-ovarian system (HPO system) of herbal medicine

Menstrual irregularity is an endocrinal disorder that is often observed in females of reproductive age. Many researchers have vigorously investigated the etiology and pathogenesis of the menstrual irregularity and the pharmacological action of several agents, and as a result, the mechanisms underlying menstrual irregularity have been gradually clarified. Namely, menstrual cycle is regulated by the hypothalamic-pituitary-ovarian system (HPO system). Secretory dysfunction of the GnRH, FSH, LH and E2, as well as abnormalities of those receptor induce dysfunction of the HPO system, leading to menstrual irregularity, such as amenorrhea.

It is thought that the therapeutic strategy of Western Medicine is not adequate to treat menstrual irregularity, even though variable regimens have been developed. Recently, it has been suggested that traditional herbs and Kampo formulae can influence the HPO system.

2.1 Single herb

2.1.1 Pueraria mirifica (a Thai herb)

Pueraria mirifica (PM), a Thai herb, contains a large amount of phytoestrogens. Estrogen-mimicking plant compounds, in its tuberous roots have been used as a rejuvenating drug in Thailand (11). However, the clinical effects of PM on lipid metabolism and the underlying molecular mechanisms remain undetermined. Previously, we examined the effects of PM on serum lipid parameters in a randomized, double-blind, placebo-controlled clinical trial, because Impaired lipid metabolism is an important health problem in postmenopausal women with insufficient estrogen. After 2 months of treatment, the PM group showed a significant increase in serum concentrations of high-density lipoprotein (HDL) cholesterol and apolipoprotein (apo) A-1 (34% and 40%, respectively), and a significant decrease in low-density lipoprotein (LDL) cholesterol and apo B (17% and 9%, respectively), compared with baseline measurements. Moreover, significant decreases were observed in the ratios of LDL cholesterol to HDL cholesterol (37%) and apo B to apo A-1 (35%). Recently, the effects of PM phytoestrogens on the activation of estrogen receptor (ER)-mediated transactivation have been determined by transient expression assays of a reporter gene in cultured cells. Among PM phytoestrogens, miroestrol and coumestrol enhance both ERα- and ERβ-mediated transactivation, whereas other phytoestrogens, including daidzein and genistein, preferentially enhanced ERβ-mediated transactivation. Taken together, PM has a beneficial effect on lipid metabolism in postmenopausal women, which may result from the activation of gene transcription through selective binding of phytoestrogens to ERα and ERβ (12).

2.1.2 Vitex agnus castus (Japanese name: Seiyoninjinboku: Not a Kampo herb)

Vitex is a deciduous shrub native to European, Mediterranean and Central Asian countries. *In-vitro* studies describe dopaminergic effects of Vitex via dose-dependent binding of dopamine-2 receptors, yielding potent inhibition of prolactin in cultured pituitary cells. The flavonoid apigenin can be isolated from Vitex and has selective binding affinity for the β-estrogen receptor subtype (13). Human studies reported inhibition of FSH and stimulation of LH secretion and presumed the hormone modulation of FSH and LH affected the downstream hormones progesterone and estrogen (14, 15). Based on current pharmacological studies and RCTs, Vitex is indicated for hyperprolactinemia - related reproductive dysfunction (16).

2.1.3 Cinnamon bark (Japanese name: Keihi)

Cinnamon bark is a major herb of the Kampo formulae: *Keishibukuryogan* and *Tokikenchuto*, which are indicated for several menstrual disorders. While several pharmacological studies have suggested anti-inflammatory properties, the mechanisms by which the herb exerts its various activities are not yet well understood. Cinnamaldehyde, a major active constituent of Cinnamomum cassia has been shown to stimulate cathecholamine release from the adrenal glands. On *in-vitro* analysis, exposure of human adrenal cells (H295R) to cinnamaldehyde increased progesterone release in a dose-dependent manner. In contrast, the release of cortisol or estradiol was not affected by treatment with cinnamaldehyde (17). Recent reports suggest menstrual distress is related to higher estradiol levels, higher estradiol/progesterone ratios (18). Therefore, these actions of cinnamaldehyde may be attributed to the clinical effects of Cinnamon bark.

2.1.4 Cimicifuga racemosa (Japanese name: Shoma)

Extracts (ethanolic and isopropanolic aqueous, Remifemin) of the rootstock of the herb Cimicifuga racemosa (black cohosh) are active ingredients developed for the treatment of gynecologic disorders, particularly climacteric symptoms (19). Drug-monitoring and clinical studies documenting experience with Cimicifuga racemosa rootstock extracts have provided a database on the effect of this herbal treatment for menopausal symptoms (e.g., hot flashes, profuse sweating, sleep disturbances, depressive moods). These studies have shown good therapeutic efficacy and tolerability profiles of Cimicifuga. In addition, clinical and experimental investigations indicate that the rootstock of Cimicifuga racemosa does not show any hormone-like activity, as was originally postulated.

2.1.5 Angelica sinensis (Japanese name: Toki)

One of the most common applications for Angelica sinensis in the United States is for relief of vasomotor symptoms associated with menopause. Such symptoms include hot flashes, skin flushing, and increased perspiration. The mechanism of action, however, is still unclear. In a randomized, double-blind, placebo-controlled clinical trial, 71 postmenopausal women received either Toki (4.5 g) or placebo daily for 24 weeks (20). There were no differences in vasomotor symptoms between the two groups, and there appeared to be no estrogen-like effects on vaginal epithelial tissue. The use of Toki alone can be criticized because traditional Herbal practitioners never prescribed it alone, but rather in combination with several other herbs.

These observations are very interesting, because Kampo formulae are water extracts, sometimes caledl "decoction", namely crude drug, which contains a great many ingredients. It is considered that the action of Kampo formula may be multi-targeted. A herbal mixture containing Angelica sinensis root, Paeonia lactiflora root, Ligusticum rhizome, Atractylodes rhizome, Alismatis rhizome, and Sclerotium poria has been reported to reduce menopausal disturbances, including vasomotor symptoms by about 70 percent (20, 21)

2.2 Kampo formula: Several herb mixture

2.2.1 Tokishakuyakusan (Chinese name, Dang gui shao yao san)

Tokishakuyakusan (root of Angelica, peony root, cnidium rhizome, alisma rhizome, atractylodis rhizome, poria sclerotium) is a commonly prescribed Kampo formula for menstrual irregularity or menopausal symptoms in woman. The action of this formula on HPO system has been analyzed *in vitro* and in several animal models. First, in the preovulatory follicles incubated in vitro, it has been demonstrated that Tokishakuyakusan stimulates preovulatory follicles before a LH surge to secrete progesterone, but Tokishakuyakusan suppresses E2 secretion by growing preovulatory follicles before the LH surge (22). However, in vivo, Tokishakuyakusan increases the concentrations of estradiol-17 β(E2), progesterone and testosterone (1, 23). These observations suggest that Tokishakuyakusan influences the HPO system. Recently, it has been reported that Tokishakuyakusan has an influence on the brain in the ovariectomized mice. Administration of Tokishakuyakusan significantly suppressed the decrease in choline acetyltransferase activity in the cerebral cortex and the dorsal hippocampus of the ovariectomized mice (24). These phenomena may explain the mechanism of action of Tokishakuyakusan on mood disturbance in human climacteric disorder.

2.2.2 Keishibukuryogan (Chinese name, Gui zhi fu ling wan)

Keishibukuryogan (bark of Cinnamomum cassia, root of Paeonia lactiflora, seed of Prunus persica or P. persiba var. davidiana, carpophores of Poria cocos, root bark of Paeonia suffruticosa) is a traditional herbal formula used in Kampo medicine in Japan. This remedy for menopausal symptoms has been approved by the Ministry of Health, Labor and Welfare in Japan. To date, there have been several studies demonstrating that Keishibukuryogan ameliorates menopausal hot flashes. The action of this formula on HPO system has also been analyzed *in vitro* and in several animal models.

It has been reported that oral administration of Keishibukuryogan may act as a LH-RH/GnRH antagonist and/or have a weak anti-estrogen effect in the rat model (25). However, Keishibukuryogan also increased the concentrations of E2, progesterone and testosterone, in vivo rat model (23). Recently, it has demonstrated that oral Keishibukuryogan administration did not affect the decreased concentration of plasma E2 and decreased uterine weight caused by ovariectomy, although hormone replacement with E2 restored them, in ovariectomized rats (3). These findings suggest that Keishibukuryogan, which does not alter plasma levels of estrogen, may be useful for the treatment of hot flashes in patients for whom estrogen replacement therapy is contraindicated, as well as in menopausal women.

Furthermore, Keishibukuryogan demonstrates several other activities such as effects on immunomodulation and microcirculation. Therefore, Keishibukuryogan is usually administered to the patients with gynecological disorders, as well as inflammatory diseases such as rheumatoid arthritis and disturbances of the peripheral circulation in Japan.

2.2.3 Kamishoyosan (Chinese name, Jia wei xiao yao san)

Kamishoyosan (Bupleurum root, root of Angelica, peony root, atractylodis rhizome, poria sclerotium, menthae herba, zingiberis rhizome, licorice root, moutan bark, gardenia fructus), a Kampo formula used to treat menopausal psychotic syndromes in women, consists of ten crude herbal preparations. The anxiolytic effect of Kamishoyosan has usually been investigated using the social interaction (SI) test in mice. Whether the effect of Kamishoyosan was due to the stimulating and/or sedating effects was examined by the open field locomotion test (26). It appears the Kamishoyosan-induced SI behavior is due to its anxiolytic effect. The unaltered results of the open field test indicated that kamishoyosan was neither a stimulant nor sedative. Furthermore, Gardeniae Fructus in Kamishoyosan and geniposide (its ingredient) play a role in the anxiolytic effect of kamishoyosan. This formula may not be effective to ameliorate menstrual disorders, but for psychotic symptoms in women.

2.2.4 Unkeito (Chinese name, Wen jing tang)

From ancient times, Unkeito (Pinellia tuber, Ophiopogen tuber, root of Angelica, peony root, cnidium rhizome, Ginseng radix, bark of Cinnamomum cassia, Asini corii collas, Moutan bark, licorice root, zingiberis rhizome, Euodia fruit) is a representative formula for the treatment of menstrual disorders, and at present, this Kampo formula has usually been administered to the patients with menstrual irregularity. The action of Unkeito on the HPO system has been clarified by several researchers (27 - 29). In vitro analysis has also demonstrated that Unkeito stimulates the secretion of progesterone from the preovulatory follicles before the LH surge, but Keishibukuryogan suppresses E2 secretion by growing preovulatory follicles before a LH surge (22). To analyze the effect of Unkeito and its components on LH-RH/GnRH and LH release in an animal model, the mediobasal hypothalamus (MBH) alone or the pituitary alone or the pituitary in sequence with the MBH from normal female rats in diestrus was perfused in a sequential double-chamber perfusion system (30). These analyses demonstrated that Unkeito induces GnRH-induced LH release from the anterior pituitary and can be used for the treatment of patients with hypothalamic amenorrhea.

3. The clinical efficacy of herbal medicine for menstrual irregularity

As described, several herbs and Kampo formula have the potential to improve menstrual disorders, caused by disturbance of the HPO system. However, it is well known that *in vitro* studies or analyses using animal models do not always coincide with the effects in humans. Therefore, we also present evidence demonstrating the effects of Kampo formulae on menstrual disorders in clinical trials.

3.1 Tokishakuyakusan

A double-blind study was performed using Tokishakuyakusan to treat primary dysmenorrheal (31). As a result, a significant alleviation of dysmenorrhea was observed in patients treated with Tokishakuyakusan compared to that of those treated with placebo, suggesting that Tokishakuyakusan is effective for treating dysmenorrhea in patients with coldness and low daily activity. This study can be recognized as an attempt to define the indications for Tokishakuyakusan using the Kampo diagnostic system (i.e., low vigor, coldness and blood stasis in patients with dysmenorrheal). Since it is important to reduce the use of analgesics for pain relief, continued studies are expected, to determine whether Tokishakuyakusan is also effective for patients not responding to analgesics.

Another clinician has reported an antidysmenorrhea therapy using a cyclic regimen of Shakuyakukanzoto and Tokishakuyakusan, in which the herbs are administered alternately within the menstrual cycle (32). In 12 dysmenorrhea patients treated with the

Shakuyakukanzoto and Tokishakuyakusan cyclic therapy, 9 patients ovulated as determined by biphasic changes in basal body temperature patterns, suggesting that the "cyclic therapy" can be a conservative antidysmenorrhea therapy for endometriotic and adenomyotic patients who desire pregnancy.

3.2 Keishibukuryogan

Keishibukuryogan is the most common choice among complementary medicines for treatment of menstrual disorders in Japan. This formula is used to improve various signs and symptoms of endometriosis without decreasing serum estradiol levels or causing menstrual disorders. There is the examination and comparison between the effects of Keishibukuryogan and danazol on anti-endometrial humoral immunity in humans (33). Absorption tests of nonspecific antibodies using cervical cancer cells or ovarian cancer cells demonstrated that endometriotic patients had higher levels of endometrium-specific autoantibodies than healthy women without endometriosis. IgM fractions from endometriotic patients and healthy women differed in their effect on growth of endometrial adenocarcinoma cells. Therapy with Keishibukuryogan but not danazol therapy, gradually decreased the tissue-specific anti-endometrial IgM antibody levels, indicating that tissue-specific anti-endometrial IgM may be a useful therapeutic marker for endometriotic patients treated with Keishibukuryogan and that endometrial tissue-specific immune disorders play specific roles in the pathogenesis or development of endometriosis in humans.

3.3 Kamishoyosan

Although Kamishoyosan is a common Kampo formula for menopausal disorders such as psychological or vasomotor symptoms, there are few reports demonstrating the clinical efficacy of Kamishoyosan for menstrual irregularities (34).

It has been demonstrated that 30 patients with premenstrual dysphoric disorder (PMDD) were treated with Kamishoyosan for six menstrual cycles and 19 patients (63.3%) had >50% improvement in the total score on the Hamilton Depression Rating Scale (HAM-D) Scale in the late luteal phase, and 14 patients (46.7%) went into remission (35). Regarding the mechanism of action of Kamishoyosan, studies were conducted to compare the effects on serum cytokine concentrations of paroxetine, a selective serotonin re-uptake inhibitor, and kamishoyosan (36, 37). In 76 women with psychological symptoms such as anxiety and mild depression as menopausal symptoms, Greene's total scores in both women treated with paroxetine and in women treated with kamishoyosan decreased significantly. The serum IL-6 concentration in women treated with paroxetine decreased significantly. Serum concentrations of IL-8, IL-10, macrophage inflammatory protein (MIP)-1β and monocyte chemoattractant protein-1 in women treated with paroxetine decreased significantly. However, serum IL-6 concentration in women treated with kamishoyosan decreased significantly, but other serum concentrations did not change significantly. Based on the above findings, a decrease in IL-6 concentration may be involved in the action mechanisms of both paroxetine and kamishoyosan in women with psychological symptoms.

In conclusion, Kamishoyosan may be a useful agent to alleviate psychological symptoms in menopausal woman, but not for menstrual irregularities.

3.4 Unkeito

Unkeito is one of the agents in which its action on the HPO system was analyzed and several clinical trials were previously carried out. There is a representative report demonstrating the improvement of gonadotropin and estradiol secretion in either hyper- or hypo-functioning anovulatory women (38). In patients with amenorrhea, ovulation occurred in 61.3% and 66.7% of patients with first-grade amenorrhea, and in 27.3% and 22.4% of patients with second-grade amenorrhea, respectively. In these patients, 8 weeks of treatment with Unkeito induced a significant increase in plasma FSH, LH and estradiol levels in hyper- (robust) and hypo- (asthenia) functioning patients with first- and second-grade amenorrhea. There were no significant differences in the rates of change in these hormones between hyper- and hypo-functioning patients. Recently, it has been demonstrated that Unkeito increases peripheral blood flow, especially in the lower extrimities, and decreases blood flow in the upper body, in contrast, there was no difference in circulation in the upper- and lower extremities induced by vitamin E (39). Furthermore, the effects of Unkeito on the serum levels of several cytokines have also been reported (40).

4. The current topics concerning Kampo therapeutic strategy for menstrual disorders

Currently a greater proportion of the women diagnosed with breast cancer develop estrogen-deficiency symptoms compared to that in the recent past due to advances in approaches to breast cancer treatment (41). All premenopausal breast cancer patients receiving chemotherapy are at risk of the developing chemotherapy-induced amenorrhea (CIA) (41). In these patients, menopausal symptoms must be more serious than amenorrhea. Further, women with ER-positive breast cancers face additional risks and approximately 60% of cancers are ER-positive (42). These patients are not able to be treated with hormone replacement therapy (HRT). Therefore, there are no treatments to control menopausal symptoms in premenopausal patients with breast cancer. We have reported that Nyoshinsan, a Kampo formula, may be useful and a safe agent to treat estrogen-deficiency symptoms in breast cancer survivors, since managing estrogen-deficiency symptoms in breast cancer survivors remains problematic (43).

We considered treatment with Nyoshinsan for 6 premenopausal breast cancer survivors from the Department of Breast Surgery in our hospital who consulted the Department of Japanese Oriental Medicine postoperatively because of menopausal symptoms. As an endpoint, we determined the incidence of postmenopausal symptoms such as hot flashes, sweating, anxiety and depression, and measured the severity of these symptoms using a visual analogue scale (VAS). In addition, we assessed the serum level of estradiol (E2). Their menopausal symptoms were mainly vasomotor symptoms such as hot flashes and sweating, and mental symptoms such as sleeping disorder and depression, but not skeletal muscle symptoms such as shoulder stiffness. In five of the 6 patients, the Nyoshinsan treatment resulted in a noticeable alleviation of menopausal symptoms without adverse effects; one patient reported that her symptoms did not change. Changes in the serum levels of E2 are shown in Figure 1. The serum E2 levels in five patients did not change, but there was an increase in the serum E2 level in one patient, who was successfully treated with Nyoshinsan. In this patient, the administration of Nyoshinsan was discontinued and her serum E2 level decreased. A representative patient with premenopausal breast cancer who was successfully treated with Nyoshinsan for estrogen-deficiency symptoms that were induced postoperatively by adjuvant chemotherapy is also presented (Figure 2). Nyoshinsan resulted in the relief of severe menopausal symptoms such as hot flashes, fatigue, and anxiety. Furthermore, serum levels of E2 and FSH did not change from the baseline. Nyoshinsan may be a useful and safe agent to treat estrogen-deficiency symptoms in breast cancer survivors, because managing estrogen-deficiency symptoms in these patients remains problematic.

These observations demonstrate that Kampo formulae may alleviate climacteric symptoms by an action that differs from E2-like effects of folk medicines, such as *Pueraria mirifica or Vitex agnus castus.*

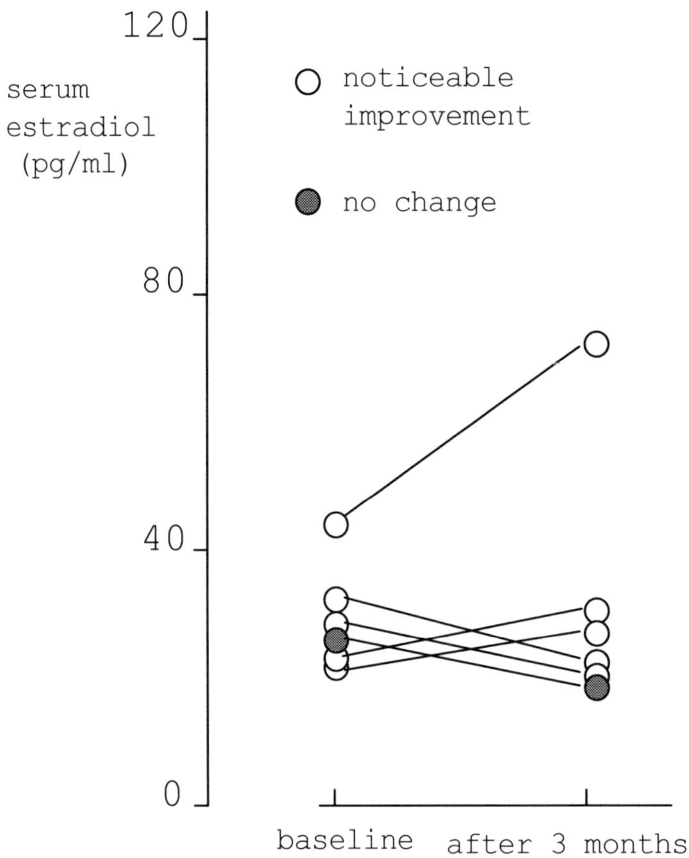

Fig. 1. Changes in the serum levels of estradiol (E2) during treatment with Nyoshinsan/TJ-67. In five patients, the E2 level did not change, while one patient showed an increase in the serum level of E2. Open circles, patients with noticeable improvement; closed circle, one patient without improvement.

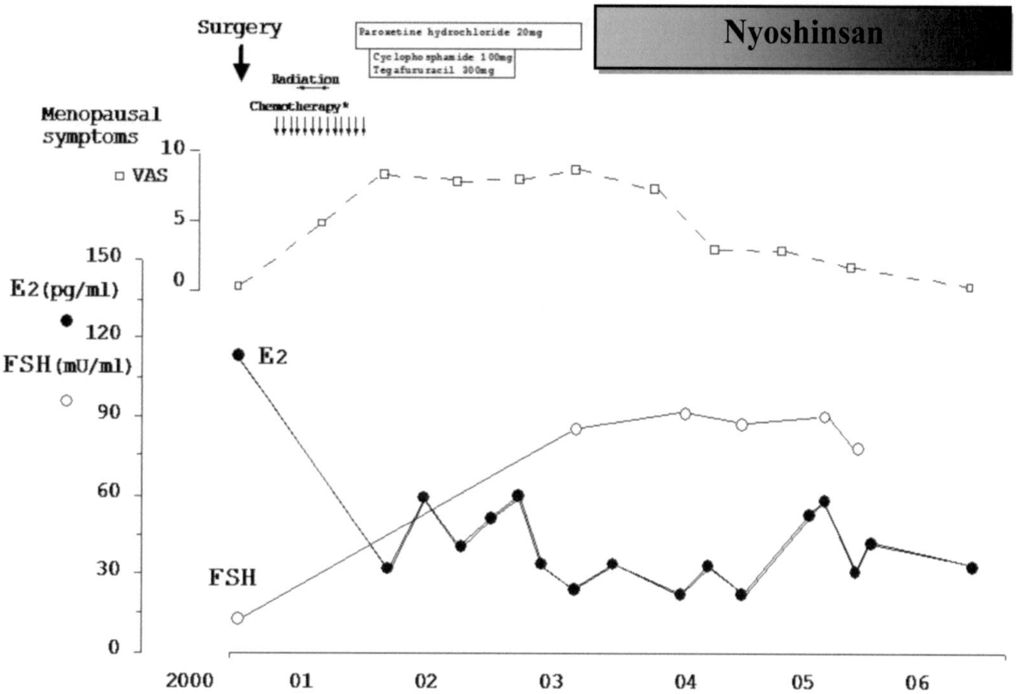

Fig. 2. Clinical course in representative patient described in the case report. The oral administration of Nyoshinsan resulted in the relief of severe menopausal symptoms such as hot flashes, fatigue, and anxiety. Serum levels of E2 and follicle-stimulating hormone (FSH) did not change from the baseline values. VAS, Visual analogue scale; chemotherapy*, cyclophosphamide 300 mg, pirarubicin hydrochloride 45 mg, and 5-fluorouracil 750 mg.

5. Conclusion

Actions on the HPO system and the clinical efficacy of traditional herbal medicine are being clarified. Traditional herbs possess unique functions that are different from those of pure chemical compounds. It has been expected that traditional herbs will become interestingly applicable to the treatment of menstrual irregularities, such as amenorrhea.

6. References

[1] Usuki S, Kotani E, Kawakura Y, Sano M, Katsura Y, Kubo T. Tokishakuyakusan effect on DNA polymerase alpha activity in relationship to DNA synthesis before and/or after the LH/FSH surge in rats. Am J Chin Med. 1995; 23:231-42.

[2] Usuki S. Effects of hachimijiogan, tokishakuyakusan, keishibukuryogan, ninjinto and unkeito on estrogen and progesterone secretion in preovulatory follicles incubated in vitro. Am J Chin Med. 1991; 19:65-71.

[3] Noguchi M, Ikarashi Y, Yuzurihara M, Kase Y, Watanabe K, Plotnikoff GA, Takeda S, Aburada M. Skin temperature rise induced by calcitonin gene-related peptide in gonadotropin-releasing hormone analogue-treated female rats and alleviation by Keishi-bukuryo-gan, a Japanese herbal medicine. Life Sci. 2005; 76: 2079-90.

[4] Okamura S, Sawada Y, Satoh T, Sakamoto H, Saito Y, Sumino H, Takizawa T, Kogure T, Chaichantipyuth C, Higuchi Y, Ishikawa T, Sakamaki T. Pueraria mirifica phytoestrogens improve dyslipidemia in postmenopausal women probably by activating estrogen receptor subtypes. Tohoku J Exp Med. 2008; 216:3 41-51.

[5] Cherdshewasart W, Sriwatcharakul S. Metabolic activation promotes estrogenic activity of the phytoestrogen-rich plant. Maturitas. 2008; 59: 128-36

[6] Haimov-Kochman R, Brzezinski A, Hochner-Celnikier D. Herbal remedies for menopausal symptoms: are we cautious enough? Eur J Contracept Reprod Health Care. 2008; 13: 133-7.

[7] Mantani N, Hisanaga A, Kogure T, Kita T, Shimada Y, Terasawa K. Four cases of panic disorder successfully treated with Kampo (Japanese herbal) medicines: Kami-shoyo-san and Hange-koboku-to. Psychiatry and Clinical Neurosciences 2002; 56: 617-620

[8] Tatsumi T, Kogure T. The possibirity of serial Determination of PAC/PRA for a Useful Maker of Pseudoaldsteronism. J. Traditional Medicine 2008: 25: 119-21

[9] Kogure T, Tatsumi T, Oku Y. Edematous erythema at the hands and feet probably caused by the traditional herb "radix astragali". Integr Med Insights. 2011; 6:1-5

[10] Mantani N, Kogure T, Sakai S, Goto H, Shibahara N, Kita T, Shimada Y, Terasawa K. Incidence and clinical features of liver injury related to Kampo (Japanese herbal) medicine in 2,496 cases between 1979 and 1999: problems of the lymphocyte transformation test as a diagnostic method. Phytomedicine. 2002; 9: 280-7.

[11] Ingham T, Tahara S, Pope GS. Chemical components and pharmacology of the rejuvenating plant pueraria mirifica. In Pueraria, edited by WM Keung. Taylor & Francis, London & New York, pp.97-118

[12] Okamura S, Sawada Y, Satoh T, Sakamoto H, Saito Y, Sumino H, Takizawa T, Kogure T, Chaichantipyuth C, Higuchi Y, Ishikawa T, Sakamaki T. Pueraria mirifica phytoestrogens improve dyslipidemia in postmenopausal women probably by activating estrogen receptor subtypes. Tohoku J Exp Med. 2008; 216: 341-51.

[13] Wuttke W, Jarry H, Christoffel V, et al. Chaste tree 7. (Vitex agnus-castus) - pharmacology and clinical indications. Phytomedicine 2003;10:348-357.

[14] Boon H, Smith M. 12. The Botanical Pharmacy: The Pharmacology of 47 Common Herbs. Kingston, ON: Quarry Press, Inc.; 1999; 76-81.

[15] No authors listed. 13. British Herbal Pharmacopeia: 1996. 4th ed. Exeter, UK: British Herbal Medicine Association; 1996; 19-20.

[16] Milewicz A, Gejdel E, Sworen H, et al. 20. Vitex agnus castus extract in the treatment of luteal phase defects due to latent hyperprolactinemia. Results of a randomized placebo-controlled double-blind study. Arzneimittelforschung 1993; 43: 752-6.

[17] Iwaoka Y, Hashimoto R, Koizumi H, Yu J, Okabe T. Selective stimulation by cinnamaldehyde of progesterone secretion in human adrenal cells. Life Sci. 2010; 86: 894-8.

[18] Fox HC, Hong KA, Paliwal P, Morgan PT, Sinha R. Altered levels of sex and stress steroid hormones assessed daily over a 28-day cycle in early abstinent cocaine-dependent females. Psychopharmacology (Berl). 2008; 195: 527-36

[19] Liske E. Therapeutic efficacy and safety of Cimicifuga racemosa for gynecologic disorders. Adv Ther. 1998; 15: 45-53.

[20] Hirata JD, Swiersz LM, Zell B, et al. Does dong quai have estrogenic effects in postmenopausal women? A double-blind, placebocontrolled trial. Fertil Steril 1997; 68: 981-6.
[21] Chang HM, But PP. Pharmacology and Application of Chinese Material Medica, Vol 1. Singapore: World Scientific; 1987:489-505.
[22] Usuki S. Effects of hachimijiogan, tokishakuyakusan, keishibukuryogan, ninjinto and unkeito on estrogen and progesterone secretion in preovulatory follicles incubated in vitro. Am J Chin Med. 1991; 19:65-71.
[23] Usuki S. Effects of tokishakuyakusan and keishibukuryogan on steroidogenesis by rat preovulatory follicles in vivo. Am J Chin Med. 1990;18:149-56.
[24] Toriizuka K, Hou P, Yabe T, Iijima K, Hanawa T, Cyong JC. Effects of Kampo medicine, Toki-shakuyaku-san (Tang-Kuei-Shao-Yao-San), on choline acetyltransferase activity and norepinephrine contents in brain regions, and mitogenic activity of splenic lymphocytes in ovariectomized mice. J Ethnopharmacol. 2000; 71: 133-43.
[25] Sakamoto S, Kudo H, Kawasaki T, Kuwa K, Kasahara N, Sassa S, Okamoto R. Effects of a Chinese herbal medicine, keishi-bukuryo-gan, on the gonadal system of rats. J Ethnopharmacol. 1988; 23: 151-8.
[26] Toriizuka K, Kamiki H, Ohmura NY, Fujii M, Hori Y, Fukumura M, Hirai Y, Isoda S, Nemoto Y, Ida Y. Anxiolytic effect of Gardeniae Fructus-extract containing active ingredient from Kamishoyosan (KSS), a Japanese traditional Kampo medicine. Life Sci. 2005; 77: 3010-20
[27] Ushiroyama T, Tsubokura S, Ikeda A, Ueki M. The effect of unkei-to on pituitary gonadotropin secretion and ovulation in anovulatory cycles of young women. Am J Chin Med. 1995; 23: 223-30.
[28] Koyama T, Ohara M, Ichimura M, Saito M. Effect of Japanese kampo medicine on hypothalamic-pituitary-ovarian function in women with ovarian insufficiency. Am J Chin Med. 1988; 16:47-55.
[29] Koike K, Zhang ZX, Sakamoto Y, Miyake A, Inoue M. Evidence that folliculo-stellate cells mediate the inhibitory effect of Japanese kampo medicine, unkei-to, on growth hormone secretion in rat anterior pituitary cell cultures. Am J Reprod Immunol. 1998; 39: 217-22.
[30] Tasaka K, Miyake A, Ohtsuka S, Yoshimoto Y, Aono T, Tanizawa O. Stimulatory effect of a traditional herbal medicine, Unkeito on LH-RH release. Nippon Sanka Fujinka Gakkai Zasshi. 1985; 37:2821-6. Japanese.
[31] Kotani N, Oyama T, Sakai I, Hashimoto H, Muraoka M, Ogawa Y, Matsuki A. Analgesic effect of a herbal medicine for treatment of primary dysmenorrhea--a double-blind study. Am J Chin Med. 1997; 25: 205-12.
[32] Tanaka T. A novel anti-dysmenorrhea therapy with cyclic administration of two Japanese herbal medicines. Clin Exp Obstet Gynecol. 2003; 30:95-8.
[33] Tanaka T, Umesaki N, Mizuno K, Fujino Y, Ogita S. Anti-endometrial IgM autoantibodies in endometriotic patients: a preliminary study. Clin Exp Obstet Gynecol. 2000; 27: 133-7.
[34] Kimura Y, Takamatsu K, Fujii A, Suzuki M, Chikada N, Tanada R, Kume Y, Sato H. Kampo therapy for premenstrual syndrome: efficacy of Kamishoyosan quantified using the second derivative of the fingertip photoplethysmogram. J Obstet Gynaecol Res. 2007; 33: 325-32.

[35] Yamada K, Kanba S. Effectiveness of kamishoyosan for premenstrual dysphoric disorder: open-labeled pilot study. Psychiatry Clin Neurosci. 2007; 61: 323-5.
[36] Yasui T, Yamada M, Uemura H, Ueno S, Numata S, Ohmori T, Tsuchiya N, Noguchi M, Yuzurihara M, Kase Y, Irahara M. Changes in circulating cytokine levels in midlife women with psychological symptoms with selective serotonin reuptake inhibitor and Japanese traditional medicine. Maturitas. 2009; 62: 146-52.
[37] Yasui T, Matsui S, Yamamoto S, Uemura H, Tsuchiya N, Noguchi M, Yuzurihara M, Kase Y, Irahara M. Effects of Japanese traditional medicines on circulating cytokine levels in women with hot flashes. Menopause. 2011; 18: 85-92.
[38] Ushiroyama T, Hosotani T, Yamashita Y, Yamashita H, Ueki M. Effects of Unkei-to on FSH, LH and estradiol in anovulatory young women with hyper- or hypo-functioning conditions. Am J Chin Med. 2003; 31: 763-71.
[39] Ushiroyama T, Sakuma K, Nosaka S. Comparison of effects of vitamin E and wen-jing-tang (unkei-to), an herbal medicine, on peripheral blood flow in post-menopausal women with chilly sensation in the lower extremities: a randomized prospective study. Am J Chin Med. 2006; 34: 969-79.
[40] Burns JJ, Zhao L, Taylor EW, Spelman K. The influence of traditional herbal formulas on cytokine activity. Toxicology. 2010; 278: 140-59.
[41] Seidman AD. Systemic treatment of breast cancer. Two decades of progress. Oncology 2006; 20: 983-90
[42] Minton SE, Munster PN. Chemotherapy induced amenorrhea and fertility in women undergoing adjutant treatment for breast cancer. Cancer Control 2002; 9: 466-72
[43] Kogure T, Ito K, Sato H, Ito T, Oku Y, Horiguchi J, Takeyoshi I, Tatsumi T. Efficacy of Nyoshinsan/TJ-67, a traditional herbal medicine, for menopausal symtoms following surgery and adjuvant chemotherapy for premenopausal breast cancer. Int J Clin Oncol. 2008; 13: 185-9.